FOREVER TAKE MY HAND

Iris Therese Smith Reid

ARTHUR H. STOCKWELL LTD
Torrs Park, Ilfracombe, Devon, EX34 8BA
Established 1898
www.ahstockwell.co.uk

By the same author:
    Dementia Poems
    Poems of Devotion and Commotion

ISBN 978-0-7223-4796-6
Printed in Great Britain by
Arthur H. Stockwell Ltd
Torrs Park   Ilfracombe
Devon EX34 8BA

CONTENTS

PART ONE

WAR BABIES: THROUGH THE EYES OF A CHILD

Prologue

My best friend and I are playing, skipping on the front with our street friends – they are our learners and teachers, our saviours. They are older than us and they know best, so we look up to them. They teach us their games and street songs. We are safe with them; they know everything.

Suddenly – silence. The skipping and singing stop. We are like statues. Our hearts have stopped beating. We are listening. The sirens are sounding the 'all alert'.

We are getting ready to run for our lives – to bolt for the safety of our shelters. We hear the droning of aeroplane engines. They are back again, getting nearer. We are white and full of fear. They are coming over to drop their bombs on us, coming to kill or gas us. The bogeymen.

We take what we think might be the last look at our friends – is this goodbye? Will we be seeing them ever again?

Then a voice breaks the silence. A street boy, a trusted friend. "It's ours! It's OK, it's a friendly." He knows the sound of every engine, be it friend or foe.

We hesitate, give a sigh of relief. The sirens give the all-clear. We can breathe again. We're safe – alive. We all carry on with our skipping game for the umpteenth time, until the next time: 'Pittatty-pattatty on your shoulders, pittatty-pattatty on your shoulders, you will be my master.'

A new war has started, we hear from the news,
Hitler's gone crazy. He is gassing all Jews,
Shooting the Gypsies, cleansing their race
For he only wants fair hair for his new human race.
He has taken most of Europe, but he wants all the world,
So his next stop is Britain, which he says he can win.
But he doesn't know Britain, they will never give in,
They will fight for their country, they will fight for their king,
They will fight for their children, they will fight for their kin.
Britain and her Allies are seeking to plot –
He cannot have the rest of the world, we must make him stop.
Hit so it hurts him, let him feel the pain,
Destroy all his homeland, destroy all within.
Use all of our bombs, let's give him the lot.
So next stop Berlin, give everything we've got.
So they bombed and they bombed till Berlin was a crater,
But carried on bombing until finding out later
Hitler was dead.
He committed suicide – he shot himself in the head.

Memories

They say that babies never remember, but I do. I was eighteen
months old when my mother put me in a canvas box and the lid
was closed on me. It was a baby's gas mask.

I remember good times, I remember bad times, I remember
we got bombed out of some places where we lived. Some
would be blown to bits, others would have windows and doors
blown off so we would have to move to other places. We even
lived in the back of shops. Some houses were fixed up. One
house we had just moved out of was fixed back up and another
family moved into it. They were all killed. They had been
hiding under the same table that we had previously hidden
under when we left there because of the bombings. We were
bombed out of three houses. Some of the places we lived in
were the back of Grimsby Road, Hope Street, Bath Street and

Sidney Street, Cleethorpes; and Eleanor Street, Victoria Street and King Edward Street, Grimsby.

I ran around the streets of Grimsby, disobeying my mother, knowing I could get away with it because she had that many children to look after; so I am not perfect. The world is not perfect – that's the way life is.

My family surname was Usher. We were a big family, seven of us, three boys and four girls.

1930: Robert, blond, blue eyes.

1932: Ronald Fredrick Rix, jet-black hair, black eyes – everyone says he is the coalman's.

1935: Shirley Estel Theodora, red hair, blue eyes – everyone says she has been left out in the rain.

1937: John Edward Harvy, blue eyes, blond hair.

1938: Iris Therese (me), golden-blond hair, green eyes.

1939: Avril Dawn, red hair, blue eyes – another one left out in the rain.

1944: Sandra, red hair, blue eyes – a war baby.

So when the war started in 1939, my mother had six small children aged from nine years old to four months old, and another child was born in the war.

PRAYER BEFORE BEDTIME

Before I lay me down to sleep,
I pray the Lord my soul to keep.
If I should die before I wake,
I pray the Lord my soul to take.

Mother and Father and all us children are sat around the fire listening to the radio telling us we are at war. I'm one year old and Mother's holding my baby sister, who is five months old. Their faces are full of fear. We know something terrible is happening by Mother's actions. She is pacing up and down and crying. Us little ones start crying with her.

They gather all the family together, sit us all down and tell us all to listen to what they have to say. They tell us we all have to be prepared because we are at war with Germany and they will be sending planes over us to drop bombs on us and gas us, but our army and navy and air force will be protecting us; they will be fighting back to stop them killing us.

We would all have gas masks, to save us from being gassed.

My older brothers keep saying, "If they come anywhere near us we will kill them."

During the next few months Mother and Father, with all us children trying to help, dig a big hole in the bottom of our garden for the Anderson shelter to keep us safe when the bombs start dropping on us. I am digging the hole with them, but the lads keep telling me to keep out of the way. They mix loads of concrete, making a big den, then put an aluminium roof over the top of it, shovelling dirt and grass over the top and leaving a hole for a door. They put two iron beds in there with straw mattresses, a Tilley lamp and plenty of boxes filled with stuff. We are not allowed to play in it until the sirens sound and then we have to run straight for it, no matter where we are or what we are doing. The older ones have to make sure the younger ones are inside first because the sirens going off mean the German planes, our enemies, are coming to bomb or gas us, but we will be safe in the shelter.

If we do not have time to reach our shelter, then we have to go in the cupboard under the stairs, or under the big wooden table.

By this time we each had a gas mask and were told to keep it with us when the sirens started. My gas mask and my baby sister's were different from the others. It was a long canvas box with a lid that you could look out of on the top. Mother tried me in it one day. She laid me in and shut the lid on me. I saw her looking at me through it. I was terrified and started crying and screaming and trying to kick the lid open.

She took me out of it and said, "Don't be scared of it. It is to save you from being gassed – it might save your life one day. But you are too big for it, so I will get you one like the others have."

Then she showed the others how to put their gas masks on. They had to put them on their face covering their nose and mouth and they had a box to put them in with a strap to go over their shoulders.

They had built large shelters down most streets for people who did not have a shelter. Most people did not have gardens, so couldn't build their own if they wanted to. Everybody had to black out their windows in their houses every night at blackout time. They were not allowed to show any lights at all, so when the enemy planes came over to bomb or gas us everything was in blackness; they had no targets.

The streets were patrolled by blackout wardens to make sure no lights were showing. By now most of the young men had gone off to war. So had our father – he was a field gunner. Mother said we were not to worry as everyone believed the war would not last long and they would soon be back home. But weeks later my two older brothers also left home to be evacuated with loads of boys and girls from down our street and throughout Grimsby. They had gone to farms out in the countryside, because we lived right near the docks and the River Humber was full of fishing boats and merchant ships. Goods from the North Sea were shipped into Grimsby and Hull to dispatch all around by the railways. So we lived in a very dangerous place. Grimsby was among the first places the enemy bombed, and as we were also surrounded by many airfields close by we were in constant danger of being bombed. That is why my brothers had to stay evacuated until the war ended.

All of us smaller children stayed with Mother. We were glad because we had made lots of friends with other children down our street – Hope Street. Mother only allowed me to play out for one hour each day and I wasn't allowed to go off the front. But my best friend and I often went out of the street when we got fed up with doing handstands up against the wall. Mother did not know this because she was too busy with my youngest sister. When she did find out I disobeyed her she was quite mad at me and bounced me up and down by my hair, which she did whenever I disobeyed her. But it was worth it because my friend and I got to explore places.

One day we had gone right down to the end of our street and were playing skipping when the sirens started. Everything went pitch-black. I was petrified. We both stood there dumbfounded. My friend ran for her house – it was nearer than mine. She ran inside. The sirens were still going on and on, non-stop. I started running for my own house, which was about a dozen doors away, only it was so black I could not see where I was going so I had to keep my hands on the wall and feel my way along from house to house and door to door. I could hear the planes coming – they were getting closer. I could hear their engines droning overhead, getting closer and closer. I had nearly reached my door when someone grabbed hold of my hand, running and dragging me along. It was my younger brother. He ran me right through our house to the end of our garden and into our shelter.

My mother went quite mad at me, but this time she did not bounce me up and down by my hair; she boxed my ears, saying, "What did I tell you? It was never to go off the front, wasn't it? You could have been killed, and you could have got your brother killed also, having to find you. Anyway, thank the Lord and thank goodness we are all here together and safe."

The planes were dropping bombs and they were making a screaming noise as they were falling down around us. It seemed to go on forever, never-ending. We were all huddled together. One came whistling down, then silence. Then thump and the sound of breaking glass as windows were blown out, thuds and whooshes. We were all scared.

My younger brother said, "Mam, I think they have hit our house – I'm sure they have."

Mother said, "Don't frighten the young ones, love. As long as we are all here and safe, that's all that matters. Possessions are no good to anyone if you're dead. You cannot take them with you. And if the house is gone, it won't be the first time, will it? At least we have each other, thank the Lord."

We must have spent nearly all night in that shelter, cowering and frightened until the all-clear sounded. It was light when we all crawled out, and sure enough our house had been hit. We all looked at it, feeling so downhearted. The windows and doors had all been blown out. It seemed to be smoking and covered in rubble. We children started crying – we had lost another home.

The neighbours took us into their house. They said to Mother, "We thought you lot were goners."

Mother said, "No, I nearly went under the stairs but I changed my mind, and thank the Lord for that."

They gave her a cup of tea and us children a drink of milk, and our grandad, my mother's father, had one too. We children always called him Grandad Pom-Pom, and all through my life I never found out why.

We were taken to another house down Sidney Street, Cleethorpes. We loved it. Mother filled the bath up – it was a long tin one. She had put it in front of the nice coal fire, then all of us children had a bath in it. She emptied it by using buckets, then hung it in the wash house, which had a stone wash boiler in which she boiled all our clothes. There was also a hand wringer in there, a dolly tub and dolly pegs. That was how Mother would do the washing. She would also wash kitbags full of fishermen's sea gear. That was her way of earning a bob or two.

After we had our bath and some tea, we went to bed. Our beds were all iron with mattresses made of straw. But we never slept soundly, even though we hid our heads under the covers, because our bodies used to jump with fear all night at the slightest noise, waiting for the sirens to start.

We made new friends.

Mother said I was old enough to start helping out with the cleaning of the house, just downstairs. We all had a job to do before we could go out to play for one hour. She gave me a bucket of water and a 'redbrick', and she showed me how to 'redbrick' our doorstep. I had to put water on the step then rubbed the brick backwards and forwards over it until it was nice and red. Everyone down our street would brick their steps. Some steps were 'redbricked' and some steps were light brown. She would leave me to scrub it, then after a while she would be back to inspect it. If it was good enough for her then I could go out to play for an hour on the front.

Every day we would have to do different jobs and none of us would moan even when we were doing the hardest work. My next job was the cooker, which was built into the wall. It was called a Yorkshire fireplace and it was made of solid iron. The oven was on one side, the fire was in the middle, and on the other side was a square iron tank for boiling water in; it also heated up the iron kettle. She would leave the tin teapot on it, so she had a cup of tea whenever she wanted. She would stew the tea leaves all day. She made lovely bread, baking it in the oven, and boiled soup on the fire. So that was my next job – cleaning the cooker. First I had to clean the ashes out of the grate, then put paper and wood in with coal or coke (whichever was available) so it would be ready for lighting. If we had no wood we had to roll newspaper round and round into strips – that usually got it going. I would then put blacklead all over the oven door and grate and polish it with a blacklead brush until it shone. I hated doing that job – blackleading – as it would take forever trying to get my hands clean afterwards.

When my friends and I were skipping we would sing our skipping songs. We had different songs for different skipping. If we were skipping one at a time we would sing:

Teddy Bear, Teddy Bear, go upstairs,
Teddy Bear, Teddy Bear, say your prayers,
Teddy Bear, Teddy Bear, switch off the light,
Teddy Bear, Teddy Bear, say goodnight.

~

Jelly on a plate, jelly on a plate,
Wibble-wobble, wibble-wobble,
Jelly on a plate.

Pickles in a jar, pickles in a jar,
Ooh haa, ooh haa,
Pickles in a jar.

Jelly on a plate, jelly on a plate,
Wibble-wobble, wibble-wobble,
Jelly on a plate.

Skipping with lots of friends, we would borrow our mother's washing line, spread it across the road, a child holding each end of the line, then take it in turns to skip through it starting with one skip at a time; then two children would skip together, increasing the number of skips until they got caught by the line. Then they had to take their turn of turning the line.

Here is a song we sang while group skipping:

One Girl Guide dressed in blue,
These are the actions that they do,
Salute to the King and bow to the Queen,
And don't turn your back on the Union Jack.

One Girl Guide dressed in blue,
These are the actions that they do,
Salute to the King and bow to the Queen,
And turn your back on the big black cats.

Here is a song we sang while playing ball:

One, two, three, aleerie,
Four, five, six, aleerie,
Seven, eight, nine, aleerie,
Ten, aleerie, catch the ball.

Stan, Stan, the dirty old man,
Washed his face in the frying pan,
Combed his hair with horse's tail,
Scratched his belly with his big toenail.

When we got fed up with skipping we would get two empty cans, make holes either side and tie string through the holes. Then we would stand on the tins holding the string and clonk up and down the street. Or we would get two pieces of long wood off the 'bombies' and nail two blocks of wood on them to make stilts. Then we would put our feet on the blocks and walk up and down trying not to fall off, which we often did.

Before we got bombed out of our house in Hope Street, my brother and sister went to Strand Street School, near the docks. Mother took us one day because she had to tell the teacher that my brother and sister would not be going there any more because of being bombed out. We now lived too far away, so they would be going to a different school.

While my mother was discussing this with the head teacher another teacher said, "It's playtime; I'll take the children for a drink of milk and take the two young ones to the playground" – which was on the roof (the only school in Grimsby to have a playground on its roof). So we had a small drink of milk and he took us up to where the children were playing on the roof. We started walking across the playground when we heard an aeroplane come droning towards us.

Someone shouted, "It's a Jerry. Run for it!"

Someone else shouted out, "Bogeymen!"

The teacher had hold of my hand and my brother's hand and was running, dragging us along. My feet were not touching the ground. I saw some boys diving into the dustbins for cover. The teacher was zigzagging while pulling us along with him. I saw two lines of bright fire coming from the plane. I looked up and saw a window and an enemy airman staring down at us. I will never ever forget his face for as long as I live. Things seemed to stop and go in slow motion. He had a helmet on his head with flaps covering his ears. I saw his eyes staring at us through a pair of large thick-rimmed glasses. He had the look of a crazy man. He was laughing. Then he was gone. To me everything was in slow motion, even though I know it happened in seconds. I was numb with shock and traumatised.

I was screaming out in fear. I thought I would never see my mother again. I remembered nothing for a couple of days, I was that shaken up.

Days later everyone down our street was talking about it, saying that the plane had gone around Grimsby firing on schools. One of my friends who went to St Mary's Catholic School said the plane had fired on their school also. It had also fired on some bridges on the railway lines, people down Victoria Street and people in the market square. Someone asked if they got him and was told yes, he was shot down over the North Sea.

I couldn't sleep for days at a time thinking the enemy, the bogeymen and their planes, were coming to get me. I would always hide under the covers, but that never helped. My body would jump continuously throughout the night and it would be twenty years before my body stopped jumping through the night.

One day while I was out playing the sirens went. We all ran for the big communal shelter down our street. Before we reached it everything went black and searchlights started scanning the skies for planes. That was the first time I had seen the searchlights and I was quite fascinated. I watched them shining bright across the dark sky, crossing over the sky, searching. I ran into the shelter and was in there all night listening to the enemy dropping bombs and flying over us.

In the morning after the all-clear sounded and everyone came out of the shelter and houses we all looked up at the sky. It was so red! For miles around it looked like the heavens were ablaze.

A couple of nights later the sirens started again. We had all gone to bed, and we were woken up by the sirens and the sound of plane engines going over our heads. It was pitch-black. Windows were being smashed in – we could hear glass breaking all around us. Mother had hold of my hand and was carrying my youngest sister, telling us to follow her and to be careful not to tread on the broken glass. She was telling us all we had to get out and go to the Anderson shelter. Bombs were falling down and screaming all around us. We saw flashing lights in the darkness. It felt like we were being blown apart.

We made it! We got outside the house, and I was thrown inside the shelter. Mother and the rest of our family jumped in. We had all made it. We were shaking and scared, but we all gave a sigh of relief. We were alive.

Mother said to us, "That was a close call – we only just got out of there."

We stayed in the shelter until the all-clear sounded, which was hours later. When we got outside to look, our house was still standing but all the windows and doors were blown out. We could not go back into it. We were moved into a big house down King Edward Street, which was back-to-back with Victoria Street, leading on to Burgess Street. Our house was joined on to a fish house, the last house on the street – we loved it.

I found out my best friend was living halfway down the street, so I was very happy to have a friend to play with. The next day my friend and I went playing among some burnt-out houses, watching some boys searching among the ruins. They told us they were looking for gas meters to get the money out of them. We were only small, but we looked at them with disappointment in our faces.

They told us, "With them enemy planes coming over to kill us, we never know when it will be our turn. It could be our family next, so what good will the money in them meters be then? So we get on with life while we still have it."

My friend and I went to the same Baptist church, down Victoria Street, every Sunday for Sunday school. That was the day we always had a bath and would put on our Sunday best. We were always given a book or Bible for good attendance, and our mothers would never allow us to miss one Sunday. They would take us right up to the front door of the Baptist tabernacle and watch us go inside.

My friend and I were listening to a neighbour one day – my mother would call it earwigging and would box my ears for it and clear us off.

My younger brother showed us some plastic stuff that looked like glass. He said he and his friends had got it off the window of an aeroplane which had crashed. They were going to make rings with it. They told us they always went to a compound near a park where they kept prisoners of war. It was surrounded by wire. They fired their catapults through a hole at the prisoners in there. When they saw them jumping around and up and down holding their arses they knew they had hit their target and would leg it. Sometimes guards would chase them, but they never did get caught. They said they were trainspotting one day when an enemy plane started firing at the bridge near Abbey Road that they were sat on. But they had not told Mother because she would not let them out again if she knew. So we had to keep our mouths shut, and they said the next time they found some plane glass they would make us both a ring.

I remember feeling hungry most of the time and living on bread and dripping, but I loved the dripping. I always loved the taste of it and Mother always baked lovely warm bread.

We had to take Mother's tea coupons and most of her other coupons to sell to the neighbours so we could buy other food. My friend and I would go to the flour mill, near the water bridge, to buy flour. We could go around the back and get a big bag of flour for sixpence and we were told not to tell anyone else.

We all had ration books because most things were rationed, even clothes and shoes. We little ones would wear wooden clogs – my sisters and I loved wearing clogs. They looked like boots, red for the girls and blue for the boys. We girls would dance around in them. The sole was all wood and was attached to the top with brass studs. They had laces and sometimes buttons to fasten them up. We wore clogs until we started school at five years old. My brother would put brass studs round the sole of the clogs to make them last longer.

Everybody was helping with the war effort by collecting iron railings and pans. They cut most iron railings down from the front of buildings and houses, so on most front walls there were only stumps left.

One day my friend and I were playing at jumping over a wall that had all the iron railings sawn off it when I caught my knee on one of the stumps. It took a big chunk out of my kneecap. A man walking by saw what I had done – I was limping and crying with my leg covered in blood. He wrapped it up with a handkerchief and I was taken to hospital to have it stitched up. My friend brought my mother, who took me home. That Sunday I didn't feel like going to Sunday school, so I asked my mother if I could stay home, but she would not hear of it. She said I was always moaning and that hurting my knee was punishment for not wanting to go to Sunday school. I thought she was telling me the truth, so I'd better go or I would be punished.

A man used to come down our street a couple of times a week. We called him Jesus because he wore Jesus sandals and he had long hair, a long beard and long clothes. All the children down the street would sit in a circle round him while he told us Bible stories, which we all loved and enjoyed until the end of his stories when he would jump to his feet put his hands in the air and say to us, "You children have to be kind and good to others and you must believe in Jesus. If you don't believe in Jesus you will all burn in Hell's fires."

That's when we all ran away from him, scared to death. But we tried to be good because we did not want to be burnt in Hell's fires. Our mothers always came outside to give him a silver sixpence or a threepenny bit to buy himself a cup of tea.

Nearly everybody down our street had mice in their house – including us, even though Mother was always spraying DDT around. She even put it on our hair and sprayed the blankets once a week so that we did not catch nits or fleas, which we never did even though we had long hair. I don't blame them for not going on our bed or in our hair, because even we couldn't stand the smell of DDT. We would have run away from it if we had the chance.

My younger brother caught a mouse one day. He tied it on to one of his toy carts and it was running around his bedroom pulling the cart round on its back. We caught him in the act and told Mother. She boxed his ears and made him kill the mouse. He threatened us – he told us to keep out of his bedroom in the future or he would box our ears. He said we were nothing but telltale tits.

We went to bed every night with rag strips wound in our hair so that in the morning when we took them off we would have long ringlets. The only trouble with rags was we couldn't sleep because they dug into our head and hurt.

We used old rags for lots of things. We would cut them into strips, then pull each strip through a square piece of mesh, sometimes making patterns, and we would have a warm fireside rug. Everyone down our street made their own fireside rugs out of their old clothes. Sometimes we ran out of coal for our fire, so we children would take a small bag each and go on to the railway lines at the back of The Maltings to collect pieces of coke or coal that had fallen off the railway wagons on to the lines while they were transporting it to the coal yards and the docks. We would walk up and down the lines collecting it and putting it into our bags to take home so we could have a fire. One day we were bent down busily putting the bits of coal into our bags – I was singing away to myself – when suddenly in front of me I saw a pair of legs. I looked up and there before me was a bobby looking down at me. That stopped me singing. I must've jumped a foot into the air.

He said, "Well now, what are you lot up to, then? You know very well you are not allowed on the railway, don't you?" He clipped my brother's ears and said, "Get off home, the lot of you, to your mother and don't let me catch you on here again."

We all legged it smartly like, and as for me I never went with them on the line looking for coal again; but I still went on the railway with my friend to play.

My oldest sister had to go to the coal yard to get Mother a bag of coal or coke, and sometimes I would go with her. The coalman used to put the bag on the two-wheeled hand barrow then pull it down to her level so she could reach it. I would also grab a handle and we would push it home that way on the road. We had to get it up a ridge to go down an alley to reach our house, so we would come to a complete stop, but there was always a gang of workers working near The Maltings and one of them (usually the same one) would help us up the ridge so we could get on our way again.

He would always say to us, "I am going to marry one of you when you are old enough to marry me, but I don't know which one I will marry because I don't know which one to pick. You are both so pretty. I will have to make up my mind – will it be the redhead with long ringlets or will it be the golden blonde with long ringlets?"

We would both go very red in the face and carry on pushing the barrow of coal. As we travelled along they would all start singing after us and we would try not to glance back at them because they would all be grinning at us while singing the same song every time we passed them by. We would pass them on many occasions when going on errands, even when we were on our roller skates, and if they did not have to help us they would still sing after us. It was always the same song, which was:

In Dublin's fair city,
Where the girls are so pretty,
I first set my eyes on sweet Molly Malone,
As she wheeled her wheelbarrow,
Through the streets broad and narrow,
Crying, "Cockles and mussels, alive, alive, oh!
Alive, alive, oh,
Alive, alive, oh,"
Crying, "Cockles and mussels, alive, alive, oh!"
And as she grows older,
And this war is over,
One day I will marry sweet Molly Malone.

My best friend and I would play on The Maltings on a night. Alongside the railway there were plenty of warehouses, some of which were full of train wagons. We would play outside one warehouse which held wheat. It had a big iron capstan outside which pulled bags of wheat up and down, to and from the top floors. The capstan spun round and round when you put your foot on a button on the floor, so we would take it in turn to have a spin on it. The capstan looked just like the ones on the docks which the ships tied a rope on to keep them against the piers. When we got fed up with playing on the capstan, then we would play on the train wagons. We were playing in a wagon full of hay one day, and I was picking it up by the handful and making haystacks with it when I saw a stash of bandages and slings hidden under the hay.

I shouted out, "Look what I have found!"

My friend looked and said, "We'd better leave them there because these train wagons are used to transfer prisoners of war in who might be wounded and may need this stuff."

So we covered them up again and went to play on the 'bomb buildings', which were houses that had been bombed and had no windows or doors and sometimes just half of the house remained with no roof but still had rafters on. The bigger boys had tied a rope round a rafter and left it hanging there near an open window so they could swing on it right through the window and let go and land on an old mattress that they had put outside. We would copy them, and as we swung through the window would always shout "Tarzan!" as we let go of the rope.

Sometimes we would play marbles with the boys. I always nicked my brother's, and I always lost them for him. We either played on the sink top or in the gutters. I liked looking at the marbles because I was fascinated by the different colours inside them. Some were big; some were small. My friend and I called them glass allies.

Whip and top I also loved to play. I was an expert at it. I could keep that top spinning all the way up our street and back. It consisted of a long round stick of wood with string tied to the top – that was the whip. The top was also wood. Some lemonade bottles had a similarly shaped lid, which we used often for a top if we did not have a wooden one. We played whip and top by wrapping the string of the whip round the top, putting the top on the ground and pulling the string until the top spun away. Then we would keep whipping it to keep it spinning.

One night around blackout time Mother had just finished closing the curtains and blinds when the sirens started, but then the church bells started ringing. It sounded as if every church in Grimsby and Cleethorpes was ringing their bells non-stop. We could hear the foghorns going from the ships in the dock. Mother grabbed our youngest and me and told the older ones to grab all of the gas masks and run to the Anderson shelter in the street, which was not far from our house – only a couple of houses away. When we got inside nearly all the street was in there. When we were settled they were frantic, saying that we were being invaded because of the ships' foghorns and the church bells ringing non-stop. The bells were ringing all night long and aeroplanes were droning overhead, never stopping, with bombs dropping frequently.

People were saying, "If we are being invaded they would not land here by boat because Churchill has told Hitler if he tries to invade us he will set the Channel alight with oil."

Everyone was on about it all night.

In the morning when the all-clear was sounded we left the shelter reluctantly, expecting to be surrounded by Germans. When we stepped outside, there were none, but the sky was a brilliant blood red, as though the heavens were ablaze with fire. We headed for our house, all of us praying that it was still there. It was, and when we got inside Mother turned on the radio. An announcer was saying that there was a Blitz on London – they had dropped bombs on London for eight and a half hours non-stop. Mostly people's houses had been hit, and they were still bombing even after the all-clear sounded.

That night Mother said we would be staying in our own home because we were all shattered. We children were put in the cupboard under the stairs on an old mattress with our gas masks alongside us. She put another mattress under the kitchen table, which was a long, solid wooden one. She gave us pillows and a blanket, then she went under the table and told us all to sleep. But we did not sleep that night anyway as we still thought the Germans would be coming for us, to shoot us.

Planes were going over us all night, but my younger brother was telling us, "Don't worry, them planes are ours – they're friendlies." He was another one who knew the sound of the different engines.

But no matter how anyone tried to make us not feel frightened it would not work. I still had nightmares when I did go to sleep because of everything on my mind. What with the sound of the bombs dropping, the blackness, searchlights scanning the dark skies, the fear of being gassed or 'screaming-meamies' falling down upon us, thoughts of unexploded bombs, butterfly bombs whizzing down upon us then hanging on trees or from roofs! Dangers surrounded us. Houses were blown apart, and sometimes the sky seemed to be on fire for miles around. Some of our friends picked up incendiary bombs, and none of us knew if we would live or die. When some of our friends were not there, we knew they were gone. Seeing friends' sad faces because they had lost loved ones, I felt like a lost soul, not knowing if I would be the next on the list. Sometimes I felt numb – I hid under the covers hoping it would go away, trying to get a little peace from it all, but that did not help. It did not work because the war was always there. We would carry on pretending it wasn't, but it never went away. It was always there in our minds – we could never shut it out.

We would play singing games with most of the boys and girls from down our street. Even some from Burgess Street and Victoria Street would join in. We would all form a circle holding hands, with one in the middle, and we danced around singing:

Wall flowers, wall flowers, growing up so high,
All the pretty maidens, they all have to die,
Excepting [the one in the middle would call a name out] Iris Usher.
She's the only one.
She can dance, she can sing,
She can show a wedding ring.
Ee-i-addio –
Turn your back to Paddy-o.

Then we would all stop going around and turn our backs on the one in the middle. The one whose name had been called would enter the ring, changing places with the one in the middle. Then we all turned to face the one in the middle and started going round again, calling different names out so each of us took a turn in the middle.

'Dusting Bluebells' was my favourite. We would form a circle standing a foot apart, and one child would dance in and out between each one stood in the circle singing:

In and out the Dusting Bluebells,
In and out the Dusting Bluebells,
In and out the Dusting Bluebells,
Who will be my master?

The child dancing through would stop and pat the one in front of them on the shoulders while singing:

Pittaty-pattaty on your shoulders,
Pittaty-pattaty on your shoulders,
Pittaty-pattaty on your shoulders,
You will be my master.

Then they changed places with each other and the one who had been patted would dance through the circle.

Another circle game with lots of friends went like this:

The big ship sails on the Ally Ally-oh,
The Ally Ally-oh, the Ally Ally-oh.
The big ship sails on the Ally Ally-oh
On the last day of September.
My father's a sailor on the deep blue sea,
On the deep blue sea, on the deep blue sea
On the last day of September.
Ally Ally-oh, Ally Ally-oh,
The big ship sails away.
The big ship sails on the Ally Ally-oh
On the last day of September.

My Mother's Cures for Our Illnesses

Every morning and every night (except Sunday, which was bath day) we had to get washed with carbolic soap. It was a big square bar which smelt of disinfectant. After that it was a spoonful of cod liver oil – it always made me feel sick when trying to swallow it, but Mother told us we had to keep it down as it stopped us from getting sick. And it worked because all through the war we avoided so many sicknesses. Even when our friends had them, we never caught anything from them. If we got a bad chest she would put hot poultices on bandages and wrap them around our chests. It would make us sweat, but after a couple of days it made us better.

My older sister always had runny, sticky eyes, so Mother would take the tea leaves out of the teapot, wrap them in bandages and put them on my sister's eyes. She would sleep all night with them on her eyes and it would dry them up.

If we got a stye in our eye she would gently rub her gold wedding ring across it and it would go away.

Some of our friends had leg irons – they told us they had had polio.

My youngest brother was in hospital for six months with diphtheria. We all thought we would never see him again, but he came back home cured.

If we got warts we would tie horsehair around them until they fell off. Also we would rub horsehair across the wart then bury the horsehair in the garden. Some of the boys would wet a match head and rub that on the wart, and it would 'burn' it off.

I always got boils – one time I had five all at once, on my stomach near to my waist – and my mother would always squeeze them. She said she had to get the cores out of them or else they would keep coming back. She made my younger brother and my oldest sister hold me down so she could squeeze the cores out. I was screaming and kicking out with pain and nearly fainting. My younger brother stopped holding me down, and he told Mother to leave me alone. He felt sorry for me and told her it was cruel and she should leave the boils to burst on their own. She left them alone, but that night she wrapped hot poultice bandages around my waist. When she took the bandages off in the morning the boils had burst themselves, and within a week they had healed up. I got the odd one after that, but never more than one at a time. I thank the Lord for that.

My youngest sister had to go into the TB hospital with a shadow on her lung, but she was lucky: she came back home after a long time in there – she was cured.

Everyone had their toilets outside in the yard, so at night-time they would have a chamber pot under their beds so they did not have to go outside to the toilet in the dark. We children had one under our beds.

There was an old lady who lived down our street whom we called Lizzy – she was our friend, our saviour. She had no children of her own, so she made up for not having any by being so kind to half the children from down our street. If ever we were in any trouble we always went to Lizzy's house and she would sort us out, no matter what it was. One day I was walking down our street going to my friend's house, which was a couple of doors away from Lizzy's, when the Burgess Street Gang were walking past.

They started on me – pushing and shoving me along, saying, "Let's get her – she is a King Eddie. She belongs to the King Edward Street Gang!" And they punched me in the back.

I started shouting at them and crying, and with that Lizzy came out of her house.

She yelled at them, shouting, "Leave her alone, you big bullies! She is not in any gang! Be off with the lot of you before I fetch the coppers."

They all ran away laughing. She took my hand and led me inside her house. She gave me a drink and some bread and dripping and said to stay with her until they had gone. She told me that when she was a youngster she often got bullied by the children down her street until her brother gave them a good hiding, and they left her alone after that.

I went to my friend's house when they had gone and we went to play on the eeling board in the river head. There were already some children on there, but they let us on with them. There were loads of big and small jellyfish going under the eeling board, and we were all bent down prodding them with sticks. I was trying to get a massive one, leaning right over to prod it, when I fell in. I panicked because I could not swim, but a boy grabbed me and I managed to grab hold of the board. Then a couple of them pulled me back up on to the board. I dared not go home to my house – I knew my mother would go stark raving mad with me as she had threatened me to keep well away from the River Freshney and the Corporation Road Bridge. I was dripping, wet through from top to toe. My shoes were squeaking as I walked, so I went crying to Lizzy. I told her what I had done and that my mother would hit me within an inch of my life for going on the river head near to the boats and barges. She had often said it was a very dangerous place, and I had ignored her once again.

Lizzy said, "Don't worry – your mother will never know. I will dry your clothes for you."

So she dried my clothes on her big fireguard that she had round the fire and she ironed them. I sat near the fire with one of Lizzy's jumpers on, which came down to my feet. My friend kept on laughing at me in it, but it was so nice and cosy and warm.

When I was dressed we went back out to play on the front, and when I went back home my mother never noticed. Thank goodness, I didn't get my hair half pulled out of my head. I was happy.

Our transport was trams, horses and carts and Shanks's pony (which was our legs).

Mother always said to us, "Use Shanks's pony and thank the Lord that you have legs to use because poor old Bill and plenty of others like him haven't."

Bill was a man who came down our street. He had lost one of his legs in the war and he also had metal plates in his skull. He would clunk down our street dragging his leg along, and we would follow him and ask him if we could see it and he would show us. We would tap it because it looked like pottery.

He said the reason he had to drag it along was because it was so heavy. He would say to us, "Go on, then, you can touch it – it won't bite you."

We would all laugh at him. We would ask him how he got his leg cut off and he said it was a present from the Germans. And the metal plates in his skull were because of shrapnel from bombs. Sometimes several of the horrible children would mock him by walking behind him and dragging their legs and laughing, thinking they were funny, but the neighbours and my mother would tell them off, saying they should be ashamed of themselves and if they saw them mocking him again they would box their ears and tell their mothers.

My mother would always give him a silver sixpence for a bite to eat or a brass threepenny piece – it all depended if she had one, because we were poor. That is why my mother used to do the fishermen's washing for them. Every time she washed and dried their gear she had to make sure she had put everything in their kitbag, because once she had fastened it up nobody was allowed to open it. The fishermen said if they opened it before they sailed they would get washed away.

One day, before I got the chance to go out to play, Mother said I was old enough to join my sister and brother in doing the daily chores in the bedrooms. Up to now I was only doing them downstairs. So she gave me a bucket of water and a scrubbing brush and a tablet of carbolic soap and I had to go on my hands and knees and scrub the bedroom floor, not forgetting the skirting boards. Then I had to come down the stairs, washing each step on the way down. When I had finished she came and checked my work, running her finger along the skirting board to make sure I had not missed it out. I also helped her to do the washing as she had kitbags of fishermen's sea gear to get washed and dried in two days, because that is when they were going to sea again. So I pushed the dolly up and down in the dolly tub full of fishermen's jumpers. I also helped her with the wringer, catching the clothes as she pulled them through the rollers. I then asked if I could go out to play. She replied that I could after I had helped her to peg the jumpers out on the line.

I said, "Can't you get the others to help you now?"

She said, "You are always moaning, you are. A moaner, that's what you are. I should have called you Moana!"

When I finally went out to play with my friend I said to her that I was the black sheep of the family. I had to do everything as my brother and sisters always managed to disappear when there was work to be done. My friend told me that next time Mother shouted for me to do a job I should make out I wasn't there. So next time she shouted out all of our names, one after the other, I ran to hide behind the kitchen door when she shouted for me. And I couldn't believe it – my sister was there before me!

I said, "So that is why Mother never finds you lot?"

So I joined her.

Every year we all had to do the spring cleaning. We had to paint the ceilings and walls. They were all done with whitewash. The house looked nice and clean, but after a while the paint would flake and leave patches, especially on the ceilings. So at night-time when my sisters and I were lying in bed, if we could not get to sleep we would lie looking up at the patchy ceiling and make pictures and patterns out of the patches. With our imagination we made out cats, dogs, houses, castles, mountains and faces. We always made out something different every time.

The boys always slept in a big iron bed in their own room, but before our two oldest brothers were evacuated they would play tricks and games on us girls. They would set things up before we went to bed.

They would come into our room and sit on our bed and tell us ghost stories. They would say to us in the middle of the story, "The ghosts are coming to get you. They are coming up the stairs." And they would pull a string with something tied on the end of it and it would bang on each step on the way up the stairs.

We would be under the covers listening with fear.

Then they would say, "The ghost is going to open your bedroom door now." And they would pull another string, which they had tied to the door handle, and the door would squeak open.

By this time we were all terrified.

Then they said, "It's in the bedroom now." And they would touch us and say, "It's getting you now."

We girls would start screaming for our mother and crying out with fright. Mother would come running into my room and box the lads around the ears, sending them to their own rooms. Then she would show us the string that they had tied to the door handle and tell us there were no such things as ghosts, and she would leave a night light on for us to calm us down. But we would still sleep with our heads under the covers.

I liked roller skating with my friend – we would go to the shops on them. We liked the skates that had ball bearings in the wheels because we could skate faster and more smoothly on them. We would run errands for our neighbours on our skates. We would be given a penny for going on the errands, but they made us earn it. We would have to go to at least six different shops for the one penny. Then we would spend it on bread pudding, but we would only buy our bread pudding from a little shop in the old marketplace, because they always put plenty of currants in it.

We always knew how to earn a penny or two, my best friend and I, and we always shared whatever we earned equally between us. Sometimes we would be given a penny to take a bet to Bookie's Alley. The bet would be a tanner or a bob wrapped up in paper. Bookie's Alley was halfway down King Edward Street. We had to go down the alley and put the bet in a hole in the alley wall where a brick had been removed. If we saw a policeman we had to play skipping until there was no one in or near the alley. Then we would place the bet in the wall. After we had done that, the bookie's runner, whom we would call the bookie's spiv (he always had on a striped suit and polished shoes that you could see your face in and wore a moustache), would retrieve the bet and take it to the bookie's house. Everyone said the bookie was a black marketeer, but my friend and I never found out what black marketeer meant. The bookie's house would be raided by the police sometimes and shut down, but he would open up further down the street.

When we collected our penny for taking bets we would change it for two halfpennies so we could play halfpenny drop with the street boys, but we never won. We would stand in the gutter and throw our halfpenny at the wall, taking it in turns, and whoever got their halfpenny nearest the wall won everybody else's halfpenny. Those street boys made a fortune out of me and my friend.

We would collect pieces of wood from off the 'bombies', chop it into small sticks and tie them into bundles with string, then sell the bundles to our neighbours. We soon sold them because everybody had open fires. We sold them for a halfpenny a bundle and we usually made twopence each.

Mother took us out one day for a treat. We were going to see one of our older brothers, who had been evacuated to a farm out in the country. We travelled quite a distance before we got there, and when we arrived our brother came running out to meet us. While our mother went inside the farmhouse with the farmer's wife my brother showed us round the farmyard. He told us he liked living on the farm. He was the only boy there and the farmer and his wife only had one daughter; so the farmer did not want him to go back home when the war ended, and that is what Mother was discussing with them.

Our brother took us into a barn where there was a cow. He said one of his jobs was milking the cow. He showed us how to milk it. He sat on a small three-legged stool and milked the cow. The milk went into a bucket he had put underneath the cow. My younger brother asked if he could try it, so he sat on the stool to have a go. When he touched the cows udders, it let out a loud moo and kicked him. He flew off the stool and went sprawling and rolling down the gutter. He got up and, rubbing his leg, started laughing about it, and when we saw he was not hurt we girls started laughing too. We could not help it, as it looked so funny the way he flew off the stool and rolled over and the way the cow turned round, looking at him with a look that said, "Keep your hands off me!"

Next my brother took us to the stables and showed us a beautiful big white horse. It was pure white without a single mark on it and with a long mane. My brother said the farmer had told him that if he stayed with him he would be running the farm when he was old enough and the white horse would be his. We had to stand on a box so we could give the horse an apple and a pat. I stroked the horse's mane even though I was scared. My brother showed us girls how to make a corn dolly each out of the corn, then we all started chasing each other round a field until I fell into a patch of nettles. I started crying – I had never been 'nettled' before and my arms and legs were covered in small white blotches where I had been stung. My brother took me to the farmer's wife, who sat me on the kitchen table and rubbed soap all over the stings, which felt better after a while. She gave us cakes and milk, then we said goodbye to our brother and travelled back home leaving our brother there as he was staying until the war ended. We children enjoyed our day out.

One day there were about a dozen of us playing skipping down our street when we looked up into the sky and saw a couple of huge fat balloons floating about. It was the first time we had seen anything like them. The boys who were with us said they were barrage balloons, so we girls asked what they were for and why they were in the sky. They told us they were to stop enemy planes coming over our town. So we girls asked if the army were in them with their guns to shoot them down. The boys called us silly girls and we carried on skipping, but we did not find out how they were used.

There were plenty of horse troughs in Grimsby, and my friends and I always played in one down Victoria Street. They were there for the horses to have a drink from. One of them also had a little tap and a tin cup on a chain for people to have a drink. It looked to us like a little waterfall or fountain and we thought it was so pretty. It looked like it was made of pink marble. We girls wished we had one in our houses so we could have a bath in it. We would climb in it and paddle about and splash each other, but sometimes a passer-by would tell us to keep out of it as it was for the horses to drink from and not a paddling pool to play in. The boys would always get a box round the ear as we legged it back home.

Every time my friend called for me to play out, I always had to take the fireside rug outside, put it over the line and beat it with a bat to get the dust out of it before I could play with her. She would help me. My friend would beat it on one side and I would beat the other side of it, and with each beat we would laugh and say, "That's for. . . ." And then we would say the name of someone we did not like.

My younger sister did not need her pram any more – she was on the front playing with us now – so Mother let us have it to play with. My brother helped us take the wheels off it; he then tied them on a plank of wood to make a trolley, and we pushed each other up and down the street on it. When the trolley seized up, then we would use the wheels to play hoopla with. We would push the wheel along and keep it going by pushing it with a stick.

My brother would make his own catapult by using a twig from a tree and Mother's elastic from out of her bloomers. She always knew it was him! The times he had his ears boxed for taking her elastic was nobody's business.

One day I went into our house and stood there with an open mouth, gaping at my mother with awe. I couldn't believe what I was seeing – she was playing the piano like an expert. It was not our usual one. She had never played the piano in her life, and she always said she could not play for love nor money. She said she could not play a note, yet here she was playing proper music. She started laughing at me because of the look on my face, then she opened a door that was on the piano and inside was a scroll with what looked like small studs stuck on it. The scroll turned round and round when she pressed her foot on the pedals.

She said, "This piano plays itself. That scroll is the music. You push the pedals and it plays like a music box. Your grandad gave it to us so you can all play with it."

We had great fun with it, pretending to our friends that it was us playing. My friend was always on it, but I never bothered playing it. I always practised on the piano accordion; it was my oldest sister who practised the piano. My oldest brother was a fantastic singer and yodeller, and my second oldest brother played a mouth organ. We would play together at Christmas time, mostly practising together, but since the two oldest lads were now evacuated we did not play any more.

The rag-and-bone man used to come down our street on his horse and cart, shouting out, "Rag and bones!" We always wondered what he did with the bones, if he got any. We children would run into our houses and get an old jumper or frock to give to him, and he would give us a balloon.

One day he gave me a goldfish, but Mother would not let me keep it. She said, "There are enough of us having to run to the shelter without worrying about the fish."

So my friend and I took it to the park and the park keeper let us put it into the pond. On the way back home we played 'hitch a ride'. We would run after a horse and cart (there were loads of them in Grimsby taking and fetching planks of wood from the woodyards) and grab hold of a plank to pull ourselves up on it. Then we would help our friends up. The driver always slowed down for us until we were all sat on a plank, then he would make the horse go faster. When we got near the woodyard, which was near the Corporation Road Bridge, which we called the water bridge, we would all get off and sit on the bridge on a board, sunbathing or fishing. It was always full of older boys swimming when it was sunny. Some of them would dive off the side, and smaller children would get a fish head, tie string to it and throw it over the side to catch crabs. One time we pulled the fish head up and it was packed with crabs. We were all busily pulling them off and putting them in an old tin that had water in it when one of our friends who always played with us screamed out. A crab had latched on to her thumb. She was trying to shake it off and some bigger boys tried to get it off for her, but it wouldn't budge one inch. It was hanging on to her thumb for dear life, and she was jumping up and down shaking it and screaming. Then she ran home with it still hanging on to her thumb. We were all rolling over with laughter, with tears in our eyes. It was so funny! We were doubled up holding our stomachs, but we still felt sorry for her because her thumb had gone blue when we were trying to knock the crab off. When we saw her later we asked what had happened – how did she get it off? She said it dropped off when she was nearly home.

My mother always threatened to punish me within an inch of my life if I did not keep away from the River Freshney, but I always went. I thought it worth a good hiding because my friend and I always enjoyed playing there. The older boys would make a raft and when the water was high they would sometimes let us have a ride on it.

We would watch the bridge rise up to let the boats and the barges through so they could take their goods to warehouses each side of the bridge to unload. One day we made a raft and floated alongside a barge, all of us using our hands or sticks to steer the raft. Men were working on the barge and one of them threw us a large bag of peanuts. We took it home with us and shared them out with our street friends.

I always had nightmares about that bridge. I dreamt I was on it as it was going up to let boats through. I would be running up to the top of it to try to get off before it rose right up, but I had to hang on to the side of the bridge so that I did not fall off into the water, and I would hang on to it until it came back down and I was safe. My friend said she always dreamt about the same thing. She called them nightmares.

In another nightmare I would always have I was standing in the middle of the road. The street was empty – there was no one there except me and this horrid man. He was behind me, about three yards away. I had this fear – I thought he was going to kill me – so I ran to try and get away from him and he ran after me, but we were stuck on the same spot, never getting anywhere – he never caught me.

In another nightmare I always had I was falling out of bed. I was just falling, falling, falling – it was a long way down that I was falling. I dared not hit the ground because if I did, I would die. But I never did hit the ground. I would just keep falling. Sometimes I would be just going to hit the ground, thinking to myself, 'This time I cannot help hitting the ground,' but I would wake up with a bang and realise I was not falling. I was safely in bed.

In yet another dream, or nightmare, I thought I could fly. I would take off and start flying and gliding in the air. I would fly up and down the stairs. I would see my friend and she would fly around with me. We felt happy and free. We were contented while we were flying around, but we told each other we had to keep flying – we must not land, otherwise we would not be able to be free, we would never fly again, we would both die.

We would play 'knock door, run' with our street friends. We would get a length of string, tie it on the doorknob of a neighbour's house, tie a milk bottle on the other end and place the bottle on the window ledge. Then we would knock on the door. The owner would open the door to see who it was and it would pull the bottle off the window ledge. It would smash on the ground. We would all leg it, with the owner shouting after us, swearing and cussing. "If I catch you doing that again I'll box the lot of you round the ears."

We would all stand and laugh at him.

The next time we set it up on his house and knocked on the door the man did not open it. We looked at each other flabbergasted – we knew he was inside as we saw him look out of his window, so we all sneaked up and a couple of us banged hard on his window while the others banged loudly on his door.

We said to each other, "That will make him open it!"

Then we heard a squeaking noise and we all looked up to see what it was. He had opened the window of his bedroom and he threw the contents of his chamber pot all over the lot of us. We all got it in our faces.

He was laughing out loud as we were running off, and he shouted after us, "That will teach you lot a lesson, won't it? If you ever come here again you will get the same treatment!"

We all ran for a tap in the back alleyway so we could wash our faces and our hands – we stank of wee. My best friend and I never played 'knock door, run' again after that. I hated carbolic soap, but that night I could not wait to wash with it.

While out skipping in our road with about six of our friends, people were shouting at us to get out of the way and get out of the road. We panicked when we knew why they were shouting at us – there was a big brown cow running crazily down our street, heading straight for us with lots of men running after it. We all ran in all directions and the cow ran towards the central market (the market clock, we used to call it). The men went running after it. Later we were told it ended up in the river by the water bridge and they had to use a crane to get it out. We children discussed it between ourselves, saying that it was no wonder it ran away – it knew it was going to be killed. It had run away from the little cattle market beside the railway station. Not far from where we lived was a back alley which we used for a short cut to Burgess Street and the coal yard. There was a gap in the wall about halfway down which we would look through and spy on the men who killed animals there. One boy, whom we called Mad Eddie, used to ride on a cow's back and hang on to its head. The cow would run around and kick crazily about, trying to throw him off its back, just like a bucking horse. Then he would fire a small handgun into the back of the cow's head behind its ears and the cow would drop down dead on the floor. Then they would hang it up on a hook, cut it open and clean it out (steam would come out of its belly).

I would have to go to the butcher's shop to buy a 'beast heart' from him for my mother. It had loads of meat on it to feed all the family, but I never ate meat – I did not like it or the smell of it. It made me feel sick. Also whenever I had to go to the butcher's I hated it because he had loads of rabbits and hares hung up in his shop.

I loved Mother's baked bread pudding, powdered eggs and black treacle – that is when we could afford it.

Playing out in our street one day with our street friends, everyone went in apart from me and one boy who was about three years older than me. He said he was not tired. Then he took his coat off and said to sit on it and he would give me a ride, so I sat on it and he walked round and round my house, pulling me along on his coat. I was so relaxed – I had never felt so at peace. I felt safe. I felt like I was being protected. He pulled me around for ages, but it did not last. The sirens started going off and we both ran for shelter. The planes sounded right overhead, and I heard the whistling of a bomb coming down on me. I knew that sound, and I knew it would fall straight on me.

I said to myself, "Goodbye, Mam and Dad. I love you and my brothers and sisters."

Time seemed to stand still, then someone swept me off my feet and was running with me. I saw the shelter and was tossed inside. I looked up as I was falling inside the shelter and saw a man in army uniform. There was a boom and then a bright flashing light, and he stood with his arms and legs outstretched in midair. He looked like he had been electrified. I don't remember any more about what happened after that – my mind was blank for days. Weeks later, I wondered about the boy who dragged me around on his coat, but I never saw him again.

My youngest sister, my friend and I would go behind the exchange to collect coloured plastic wire out of their bins so we could make necklaces and bracelets with it. It was pretty colours – red, yellow, blue and black. We would twirl it round or plait it together. We even made rings with it. We would make peg dolls out of Mother's wooden clothes pegs, draw faces on the pegs and dress them in clothes we made out of rags.

My auntie was getting married to an American serviceman whom she had been courting for quite a few years. They took me and my youngest sister shopping; they took us into a shop which was full of toys and there were so many different pretty dolls hung up around the shop. Both of us were looking round in awe.

Then they said, "You two can pick any doll that you want. It's a present from us as we want you two to be our bridesmaids."

I picked a long raggy doll and my sister picked a short, fat pottery doll. This was the only present I can ever remember being bought for me (but we were at war).

My auntie also made us bridesmaids' dresses out of parachute silk. Mother had asked her to make the dresses so we could wear them for Sunday school and Sunday best.

We had the best day ever when she was married, and that Sunday at Sunday school we were made a sunbeam. We had to stand up in front of everyone and sing:

> Jesus wants me for a sunbeam,
> A sunbeam, a sunbeam.
> Jesus wants me for a sunbeam
> And I'll be a sunbeam for Him.

Before we went home we were given a reading book with our name on it for being a sunbeam and for good attendance.

Everyone used to say how my sisters and I had lovely long ringlets in our hair. I wasn't keen, because whenever I did anything wrong Mother would always bounce me up and down by my hair, and I would threaten her that once I was old enough I was going to cut my hair off.

My youngest brother was in the King Edward Street Gang. My friend and I asked if we could be in the gang, but they said no, we weren't old enough. We had to wait until we were seven years old. Meanwhile we had to swear an oath not to follow them or go on their territory or we would not be able to join them at all. So we had to repeat after them with one hand on our hearts and our other hand on the Bible, "We swear we will not follow you. We are not allowed to go over the water bridge. We are not allowed to go on the docks or railways."

So we swore on oath and kept it until we started school. We would not follow the gang anyway or go over the other side of the water bridge because we knew the other gangs would catapult us if we did.

My friend and I would go window-shopping and we pointed at everything we were going to buy – it would be ours when we were old enough. Nearly every shop had us fascinated. Guy and Smith's window always had the boys staring in it as it was full of aeroplanes, especially models that you could stick together and make up yourself.

One window we liked had an old lady dressed in black lace, sat on a chair rocking to and fro. Facing her on the other side of the window was an old man, also dressed in black, with little glasses on. He was also rocking to and fro on a rocking chair. Another shop was for baby clothes – it had a beautiful large pottery doll laid in a crib, dressed in baby clothes.

The butcher's shop had loads of pink pottery pigs of all different sizes. We would point at them and say, "Look, that is baby pig and mother pig, and that big one is father pig." But we did not stay looking at them for long, because we did not like the smell of the rabbits hung on his open door.

We loved Lawson and Stockdale's because they had models dressed in ladies' clothes. We would point at a dress and say that it would be ours when we were older.

I saw a beautiful blue dress with a big square sailor's collar on it and said, "That one is mine and that blue muff – they are both mine."

My friend said, "You cannot have them as they are mine – I saw them first."

Then we would argue and fight over them, and although she was a good foot taller than me I always won the fight.

She would start crying and say, "I'm never ever going to be your friend again. I mean it – not ever again. And I am not your friend now."

We would head back home, and she would walk in front of me sulking, then go into her house and slam the door on me. The next day she would come calling for me to play and everything would be forgotten. We would be the best of friends again and share everything.

Every day we would play with our street friends. We even had some friends from the neighbouring streets – Burgess Street and Victoria Street – only the ones who were round about our age, though, because, like my brother's gang, they would not let us join them because we could not run as fast as they could.

Entertainment for the War Effort

On 5 June 1943 I was nearly five years old. In two months' time I would be going to school. My best friend was already five. A neighbour was teaching us and most of our friends how to sing and dance because we were going to do a show in a hall down our street to get money for the war effort, which would be put towards buying aeroplanes needed for fighting the war. There were to be marches and parades through the streets of Grimsby – including Victoria Street, which was the street alongside ours. They would be marching all along right up to Cleethorpes. They called it 'The Wings of Victory'. There would be competitions and children's choirs in the squares and markets, shows in the schools and shows like ours, which the smaller children would be doing because we were not quite old enough to be going to school.

There was a bomber on display in a field near Louth, not far from us – my brother told us that he and his gang had already seen it. My older sister had a programme from school – she was doing drama with her class. She told us she was going to sing with the school. I had to laugh – I had heard her sing before and she sounded like a foghorn.

When we went to the hall there were twelve of us. We were to do one act a day from 7 June to 12 June – six acts.

For our first act (on day one) we had all made ourselves hula-hula skirts from green crêpe paper with a garland of flowers for our hair, and no shoes, just a flower band around our ankles. We were doing a hula-hula dance. We stood in line a foot apart and swayed our hips and hands from side to side and from front to back as we all sang:

> She wears red feathers and a hula-hula skirt,
> She wears red feathers and a hula-hula skirt. . . .

Our second act (on day two) was a cancan dance. We made cancan dresses out of net curtains with lots of layers of underskirt. We had a silk band round our hair with white socks and sandshoes. We stood in line with our hands on each other's shoulders, kicking our legs up and down in sequence while moving up and down the stage, singing as we went:

> I love the sunshine of your smile,
> I love the laughter in your eyes. . . .

For our third act (on day three) we all dressed as tramps. We put black on our face and carried a stick over our shoulder with a spotted hanky tied on the end of it. We strolled in pairs round the stage, singing together:

> We're a couple of swells,
> We stop at the best hotels. . . .

For our fourth act (on day four) there were four lamp posts on the stage with a girl standing near each post dressed in a black shiny skirt, black school stockings, a red T-shirt and a black beret. Four other girls dressed as boys, each with a kerchief tied round her neck, pretended to smoke a cigarette and walked round each girl while the rest of us girls just stood there watching them. The neighbour who taught us to sing and dance walked up and down, going in and out between us, singing 'Lili Marlene':

> Underneath the lantern
> By the barrack gate. . . .

Our fifth act (on day five) was 'How Much Is That Doggie in the Window?' On stage we had a fake window made out of cardboard on which we drew puppies with one puppy wagging its tail. We stood around this window, walking up and down, sometimes pointing to the puppies while singing:

> How much is that doggie in the window –
> The one with the waggly tail . . . ?

Our sixth act (on day six) was our last act. We all stood on the stage singing war songs with everybody joining in: 'The White Cliffs of Dover', 'It's a Long Way to Tipperary' and 'Pack Up Your Troubles in Your Old Kitbag'. Our neighbour, who had organised it, thanked all of us children and said we had done well and that they had loads of contributions for 'The Wings of Victory'. We children all loved doing it.

Then it was back to normal with sirens and bombings.

Mother always shouted to me to go to the shop for her. The shop was only round the corner, so I did not mind going on her errands, but she would send me for one cigarette at a time. I would be running to the shop five times and I could not understand why she did not buy five cigarettes at a time instead of one; then I would not have had to go backwards and forwards so many times. Sometimes she would chain-smoke – I think she lit each cigarette with each dog-end. If I complained she would tell me to stop moaning; I would be cheeky and tell her to stop smoking.

She would say, "That is easier said than done with the worries I have."

She would sit in front of the fire, poking it time and time again until she had red fire rings on her legs. Every day she would sit listening to the radio, early every morning and every night. My big sister said it was because she worried so much.

One day Mother treated us all to go and see a pantomime which was showing at the Palace Theatre, just beside the water bridge, next to the flour mill, facing the Globe Cinema. She said that because we had been so good we could also have a bag of roasted chestnuts. A man would sell them outside the cinemas and picture houses. He had a handcart with a square iron oven with chestnuts roasting on the top of the coals. We all got a bag each to eat inside, then we had to climb a load of stairs to get to the gods, as it was called. In the interval some of the boys would lean over the balcony and throw things down on the people's heads, trying to hit those with bald heads who were sitting below. If they got caught they would be thrown out and banned.

We enjoyed the show and my sister and brother took us home. On the way we met the organ grinder, as we would call him. He had a fancy box on a handcart. It had a handle on it, and when he turned it round a lot of little doors would open and it would play a tune, then wooden dolls came dancing and turning round just like a cuckoo clock. My brother gave him a brass threepenny bit and he would play it again for him.

A few nights later we were all tucked up in bed (I was fast asleep) when the sirens started. I jumped out of bed and sneaked a look out of the window. Flares were being dropped.

Mother came into the bedroom shouting out, "We haven't got time to run to the shelter. Get under the table and into the cupboard under the stairs."

As we did this, the planes were already dropping bombs.

Hearing the sounds of the bombs dropping, my brother said, "Oh, well, this is our lot – I think we have had our lot."

When the raid had stopped, we went outside into the street and we could not believe our eyes. The whole of Grimsby seemed to be on fire. Lots of places were still burning. Our side of the street was safe, but behind us The Maltings was burnt out. There were butterfly bombs spread on rooftops. I said how pretty they looked – they were yellow and green – and my brother said not to touch any as there were not only butterfly bombs around; there were also antipersonnel bombs and incendiaries lying about. Some of Victoria Street was rubble, and I could see people digging through it. There were still small flashes and bumps as explosives went off, screeching of shrapnel and people screaming. My mother was standing talking to some neighbours. I ran down the street looking for my friend – she was all right. We both went down the street to the market clock, where people had been laid around on the ground.

An army man and a policeman said to us, "Is your house still standing?"

We said, "Yes."

Then the army man said to the policeman, "Get them out of here – they don't want to see this."

We ran back home.

Days later, when we were in bed, the bombings started again. Mother had kept us in – we had not been allowed to go out at all. My brother told us we could not because there were too many small unexploded bombs still outside, and so many people had been killed – many of them down our street.

We would also be in the way of people trying to clear up, so we had not been out for weeks. We had been bombed again, and this time it was as if the whole of Grimsby had been blown up. Weeks later I met my friend at Sunday school and we walked back home together talking about it. We saw St James Church had been bombed, and we saw a huge bomb stuck in the middle of Victoria Street.

It was months later that we both started school. We should have gone to school when we were five, but because of all the clearing-up we were both nearly six by this time, and when we met our friends on a night after school we found out we had lost one. She was one of our friends from a street near us that used to come and play skipping with us. So when we all got together we made a pact: for every friend or relation we had lost, a child would sit in the middle of the ring and the rest would walk around singing 'The Ally Ally-oh'. It started off with five sitting in the middle – most had lost their fathers.

We were lucky, my friend and I, because we were in the same class at school. The school was right at the top of our street facing the docks. It was called Victoria Street School, but it stretched into King Edward Street so some of us little ones called it King Edward Street School. We did not have far to go to school. Our teacher was nice and we liked him, but everyone called him Pocket Balls (not to his face) because he always wiggled his hand in his pocket.

I was in trouble on my first day because I kept forgetting to call him sir, so he made me stand in the corner of the room with my back to the class for half an hour. I did not mind this one bit because I could see out of the window on to the docks, so I was watching the ships and dock workers unloading. I could have stayed watching them all day.

At home time we were given a jar of sweet cocoa to take home to our mothers. On the way home my friend and I opened it and tasted it. We could have eaten the lot. We had never tasted anything so sweet. It was good.

Another teacher we called Hitching Back, because he always scratched his back by rubbing it up and down the door frame.

My friend and I detested the teacher who took us for PT in the hall because he would make us do handstands up the wall; then he would walk by us and put his hand on the top of our legs, telling us to straighten them. My friend and I discussed what we would do about it and the next time we had PT and he told us to do handstands just sat down on the floor with our legs and arms crossed, watching him. As he walked up to us we just sat there and glared at him defiantly. He glared back but never said a word to either of us, and from then on we always refused to do handstands as we knew he would not say anything to us.

Coming home from school one day, we saw a barrage balloon in the sky and said to the boys, "Look, a barrage balloon!"

They replied, "That is not a barrage balloon; it is a Zeppelin. The difference is that a Zeppelin is long and thin and a barrage balloon is shorter and fatter."

We said, "I bet that Zeppelin is full of Germans with bombs!" The boys just laughed.

A couple of days later the radio announced that a Zeppelin had been over and dropped some bombs on a town. It had wanted to drop the bombs on London, but had been blown off course. I told Mother we had seen it one day. She laughed.

I thought because I was a schoolgirl I wouldn't have to do any chores now. How wrong was I! I still had to do them before I could go out for my hour playing on the front. So I was moaning about it and Mother said, "All right, for moaning you are not going out at all. You can stay in."

I wished I had not moaned as staying in meant after we did our chores we would sit round the fire listening to the radio, and all we ever heard on that was what was happening with the war. But that night we were lucky: a lady told us a story and at the end of it she said, "Goodnight, children, wherever you are." So we went to bed feeling happy. But all we heard all night were planes droning on and on, going overhead. We never heard the sirens, so we knew they were friendlies. Some sounded like big bombers. So my oldest sister and I lay chatting and making pictures out of the patches left by the whitewash flakes on the ceiling. Before she went to sleep she said to me that she hated the war and was sick to death of it and that poor Mother was sick with worry and frightened for the safety of all the children, not just hers.

At school one of the boys got the cane in front of the class for being cheeky to our teacher and for dipping my hair in his inkwell. All of us girls got our long plaits dipped in the boys' inkwells. He held out his hand, but before the cane hit it he pulled his hand back out of the way. So the teacher held his hand with one hand to give him a good whack, but the boy managed to pull his hand away again. The next time the teacher got the boy right on his fingertips, which looked more painful than whacking his hand. The boy winced and was trying not to show the teacher and us how much it hurt him. And he was still answering him back, but we could see by his face that it had hurt. He had tears in his eyes and was blowing on his fingertips trying to cool them down.

We played truant one day, 'twagging' is what we called it. My older sister split on us – she told our teacher we had been sent to school by our mothers. So my friend and I were called out in front of the class the next day.

The teacher said, "Right, you two young ladies, I shall be caning both of you for playing truant."

We both said that we hadn't, but he said, "Oh, so as well as playing truant you also tell lies. I have it from both of your mothers that you were both supposed to have gone to school. The pair of you have to know what it is to have respect for your mothers, and what it is to be disciplined." He said to my friend, "Right, young lady, hold out your hand."

She held out her hand and he caned her. She winced and glared at him, but as she walked by me to sit back at her desk she gave me a grin. Then he told me to hold out my hand, which I did, but as he swung down the cane to whack me I did what I had seen the boy do a week before: I pulled my hand away. I did it twice because I felt a bit frightened. I could see he was mad at me by the look on his face.

He said to me, "Right, young lady, bend over the desk."

I bent over the desk and he whacked me on the top of my legs. I yelled out with the shock and pain of it. Then I glared at him, trying to be brave and keep a stern face.

He told me to go to my desk. He said, "Let that be a lesson for both of you."

I sat down, but I knew I would not pull my hand away ever again. I would sooner have the cane on my hand because it hurt twice as much on my legs. I told my mother when I got home that he had caned me on my legs.

But she was waiting for me – she grabbed hold of my hair, bouncing me up and down with it and said, "That is for not going to school when I sent you, madam, so don't ever let it happen again. Remember you will always get found out – someone will always see the pair of you."

When I saw my friend she said her mother had whacked her one as well. I called my sister a telltale tit and told her that Mother had told me she had split on us.

She said, "Yes, and if you do it again I will hit you myself." She said to me I should be ashamed of myself as our mother had enough to worry about without me giving her grief.

I did feel sorry for my mother, so I ran errands for her, saying I was sorry. I had to buy some gas lighters – they were round pieces of netting which you put in a Tilley lamp. Then you would light it with a match to get a bright light. I also got four night lights, which were small, flat, round wax candles that we would put into a jar with water in the bottom and, when lit, they would give us light all night.

We stayed up late one night because there was to be a fight on the radio. My younger brother always got carried away when there was a fight on. He would jump up, punching the air.

Mother told us our two older brothers might be coming home soon. We waited weeks for them to come home, but they never did. Mother said they would not be coming home now after all as it was a false war. She was often saying that to us and we never understood what she meant by it. Some children did come home, but Mother said that was because they had come home on their own say-so as they did not like it where they had been evacuated to. But our two brothers were quite happy, so they would be staying where they were until the war ended

Five of us all sneaked into the woodyard – we called it the Woody. We would climb high up on to the top of the stacks of planks and jump from stack to stack. One day we heard a gang coming, so we all hid among the stacks. It was the older children from the Burgess Street Gang. They were firing their catapults at the stacks of timber. We watched them for a while, hoping they would not climb on to the stack we were hiding on, not daring to come out. We were all girls and they were boys much older than us, by about four years. We watched them coming closer to where we were and we were getting frightened, but a bobby started walking towards them and they all scattered, shouting out, "It's the cops." They ran in all different directions.

We scrambled down off the stack and ran for the fence. We could not run through the gate we had sneaked through because the bobby was chasing some of the boys through it. So we scrambled over the fence, I don't know how we did it as it must have been at least seven foot high, but we all made it without any trouble – and who wouldn't with a copper running after them?

But on the way back home we bumped into the same gang and they started running after us, shouting, "King Eddies!" and firing their catapults at us. I got hit on my forehead with a stone. Blood was spurting out of a small hole it made. I was taken to hospital, where they stitched it up.

My mother came and took me home. When we got in she sent me straight to bed for going into the woodyard. I had no tea. In the middle of the night my little sister and I sneaked downstairs to get some bread as we felt hungry. We lay in bed eating our round of bread and making faces out of the patches on the ceiling.

Now my friend and I were going to school, we broke our

oath to the King Edward Street Gang. They still would not let us join them, so we told them we would go on their territory whenever we wanted to. My brother said he did not want to look after his little sister in front of his mates and told me to keep away from his gang. So we went over the water bridge on our own. We would go into a shop near the bridge to buy a hot drink of cordial – it warmed us up when we felt cold and there were many different flavours. We were fascinated by the man who served us because he had a hook on one of his hands, but he managed quite well with it. And he would tell us how he lost his hand – he said it got ripped off when he jumped out of a plane. He would tell us stories of the First World War. We loved listening to his stories.

My friend and I were proper tomboys. We were always climbing. If it wasn't me getting injured it would be her.

Before The Maltings was burnt down by the bombs, we used to climb on The Maltings roof. One day we had climbed on it and were doing a dance on it. It must have been twenty feet high, and she suddenly fell through the roof. She disappeared on me!

I heard her screaming and shouting, "Help me! I want my mother. Get me out! It's dark in here. Help me! I want my mother. Help!"

I shouted back, "OK, I'm going for your mother."

I climbed back down and I ran to her mother's house and told her what had happened.

We heard her still screaming from across the road: "I'm frightened – it's dark down here. Get me out, please get me out!"

I felt like crying. I felt sorry for her. Her mother told a policeman and he and another man went on the roof with a rope to try and pull her back up through the hole she had fallen through. But the man came back down and said that it was too dangerous. He had left the policeman on the roof to try and calm her down as she was panicking. Meanwhile someone had brought the caretaker, who had a key. They opened the big doors at the front and, next thing, they carried her out and took her home. They told me she was not hurt, just bruised and mostly frightened. When the policeman came to my house he told me off, warning me that if my friend and I ever climbed on The Maltings again he would lock us both up. I promised I would not. Later we would not be able to anyway because it was bombed. That time I did not get my hair pulled by my mother; instead she boxed my ears! She said we were lucky that one of us did not get killed or seriously hurt.

But next time my friend really did get hurt. We all went on an outing with most of the children down our street. We were taken to Hubbards Hills for a treat by my friend's family. The two of us climbed a big hill, following a pathway which took us to the top. We looked down – it must have been about fifty feet high and full of trees. We had been told to keep to the pathway, but my friend wanted to slide down to each tree until we reached the bottom. I agreed and she went first. I was a bit hesitant, so she said she would show me what to do.

She shouted out, "Follow me!" Then she sat down on her bum and kicked herself off. She slid down over the top and slid to the first tree and had both feet on it.

She looked up at me, saying, "Come on, then, it is easy."

I thought the same, but before I had the chance to kick myself off she started rolling over and sliding down, hitting some trees on the way and screaming out with pain. I went back down the pathway. My heart was thumping and I thought, 'We have done it this time. My mother will kill me.' When I got to the bottom, she was just going in an ambulance. We were all taken back home.

She was in hospital for a long time, and when she came home she was still covered in bandages on her legs and arms. She used to brag about it to us street friends, but it was weeks before she was allowed to go to school or to play outside. I would play with her in her house most nights.

One night her mother left us alone while she nipped out.

After she had gone my friend said to me, "Let's go up and

play in the attic. It's all right – I always play up there. You can get all along the attics down our street."

So we both climbed the ladder and went up into her roof. When we were up there she started running along, and, next thing, she did a disappearing trick on me again – she went through someone's open trap door. I heard her scream and then silence. My first thought was, 'Oh, no, we are in deep trouble.' Then I started panicking, wondering what had happened. I thought she might be lying there dead. I was terrified by now. I climbed back down her ladder and ran like the clappers out of her house. My heart was thumping. I ran all the way home without stopping.

When I was inside our house my mother said, "What is up with you? You look like you have seen a ghost."

I said, "Oh, I have just been running."

I was not going to tell her what we had been up to as I knew she would give me a good leathering. I was too scared to tell anyone, so I kept quiet. But that night I could not sleep. I kept wondering what had happened to her, but I still said nothing.

The next day on the way to school I called for her. Her mother came to the door. I nearly had a fit! I asked if she was coming to school, and her mother said that yes, she would be going to school as she would be safer there. So I waited for her. On the way to school I asked her what had happened to her. She said that when she fell through the next-door neighbour's trap door she had landed on a bed and there was an old man in it who was very poorly. His wife took her home and later that night she told her mother he had died of a heart attack but that she was not to blame herself because he was dying anyway. She had said that her mother had given her a good hiding anyway and she would not be climbing in the attic ever again because it now had a lock on it. She said she was glad that she was back at school.

She asked what had happened to me. I said that I told my mother all about it and that I had also had a good belting, but I lied – I had not told anybody, especially my mother, because I was sick of having my hair half pulled out of my head. I hoped she believed me – we never mentioned it again.

One day half a dozen of our friends were going to the picture house. There was a matinee on, and they asked us if we wanted to go with them. We had never been to the cinema before and we told them we had no money. They said we did not need any as they would let us in. We both wanted to go, so we went with them. They told us that a couple of boys would go in and pay and we had to wait round the side for them to open the fire doors to let us in. When we arrived there, two went in and we waited near the doors. After a short while they opened them for us. We all went in and they closed the doors again, then we all sat down to watch the show.

My friend and I were excited as it was our first matinee. Our mothers had never let us go before because we were not allowed off the front. But now we were schoolgirls we went where we wanted, always following the older ones. We did not care if we got a good hiding for disobeying our mothers' orders because we thought it was worth it.

Before the matinee started a big organ rose out of the floor with a man on a stool playing it. He played a couple of tunes, then it went back down into the ground. We enjoyed the show and cartoons and then went home. We often followed them after that. Sometimes we would get caught and they would throw all of us out and ban us from going there again.

The Salvation Army would come down our street with their band, singing their hymns and rattling their collection tins. My friend and I were showing off and being clever in front of our street friends, so we were skipping around the band singing our own song that the older boys taught us, which was:

> Salvation Army, free from sin,
> All went to heaven in a corned-beef tin.
> The corned-beef tin was far too small –
> The bottom fell out and the devil caught them all.

Then our street friends thought they would get in on the act and were singing and laughing and shouting out, "Sally bummers, Sally bummers."

The band had gone silent and were stood watching us and listening. Then I nearly died – my mother had come out. I looked at her. She had daggers in her eyes and if looks could kill I would have dropped down dead right then.

She grabbed hold of me and said, "I am deeply ashamed of you being my daughter, madam. Get yourself inside – I shall deal with you later."

I shot inside, thinking, 'Oh, my goodness, I've done it this time. I'm in deep trouble now.' I watched them from the doorway, Mother and my friends. Mother was in deep discussion with the leader and my mother's face was full of rage. When they finished talking, she came inside and shut the door so I could not run. I thought, 'This is it.' I knew my mother and all of her family were deeply religious, and I thought, 'I've committed a deadly sin now in her eyes. She will never forgive me.'

She said, "Right, young lady, you and your friend have to make amends for that terrible discriminating cleverness you and your friend have carried out. I cannot find the words to say how ashamed I am of you. Your friend's mother, the leader of the Salvation Army and I have all decided that the two of you have to go to their rooms every Sunday after Sunday school for one hour to help them out in any way they want you to for four weeks, because of the way you mocked a good and dedicated group of people who only do their best to help the poor and wounded. So your so-called friends get away with it and you two have to pay the price."

So every Sunday we went and helped make the tea and wash and sweep up. After a couple of weeks they took us out on their rounds with them and gave us a tambourine each. We would sing their hymns with them while shaking the tambourines and rattling the donation tins.

When our four weeks were up they told our mothers we had paid our penance and we had made amends. We had helped them tremendously and they were sorry to see us go. We told them we wanted to stay with them, so our mothers let us. So every Sunday we went on their rounds with them and they said we could keep our tambourines, so we tied coloured ribbons on them. We stayed with them for at least six months before we got fed up with it. One of the songs we sang with them while dancing round the band was 'Jesus Loves Me, This I Know'.

My hair had grown right down my back – it was three feet long. My sister used to measure it. Mother would put an iron nit comb through our hair every Sunday after our bath to save us from catching nits. Which it did – we never ever got any. I hated that comb and the DDT that she would use on our hair. While she was putting the comb through my hair it would be full of knots. The comb would be tugging my hair and I would yell at her, "It's hurting! Stop yanking it! It's hurting me!"

Mother said, "Oh, stop your moaning – you are always moaning. I am sick of your moaning. You are a moaning Minnie."

I shouted at her, "Well you are hurting me with that comb. You are always hurting me. When I am old enough I am going to cut all of my hair off. I hate it! I hate my hair. I hate that comb."

My mother said, "Oh, so you hate it, do you? And you are going to cut it off, are you? Well, young lady I will save you the trouble."

She got a pair of scissors and cut it off right up to my ears. We were in the backyard and she threw my hair all over the floor. The sun was out and I looked at my hair lying on the ground and it looked just like spun gold lying there with the sun shining on it.

I cried my eyes out, saying, "I don't want my hair cut off – I don't want it cut off."

She said, "Well, I'm afraid it is too late now. Maybe you will stop moaning now you have got what you wanted."

I was upset for weeks after that – I could not get used to short hair.

At school one day the music teacher picked me out to be the solo singer in the choir. The others were jealous and called me teacher's pet. I always loved singing. We would go to the community halls to compete with other school choirs. I liked it also because we would have a full day out of school.

One day as we were walking to school a boy behind me shouted out, "I know who you are. You are Johny Usher's sister. I can tell by the way you walk – you are bow-legged, just like him. Where is your horse?"

My friend said, "Ignore him – they're just picking on us."

So I ignored him, but I said to her, "I'd like to know how he really knew I was Johny's sister, because he did not see my face. He was behind us and I never turned round, and he does not know Johny has any sisters. None of us have ever seen him."

She said, "It's because you do walk like him. You both have bow legs."

I just laughed at her and said, "Well, you have a big nose, the same as your brother, but he did not say anything to you, did he?"

My friend's mother had a record player, so when she went out we would play records and practise dancing to them. One certain record we had fun with was where the singer yodelled. We would hold the needle on it so he would be singing 'Yo ho, yo ho, yo ho, yo ho'. We thought that very funny, but her mother did not. She would tell us off for scratching her records.

One day we were playing hopscotch when the sky was suddenly full of aeroplanes. We got ready to run for it, but my youngest brother and his mate shouted, "It's all right, they are friendlies – they are ours."

So we stood watching them go over. The sky was full of droning as they flew overhead. We tried counting them, and we got to at least nineteen. The two boys said, "They are Lancaster bombers. They carry big bombs."

We found out days later our planes had bombed and blown up some dams with round barrel bombs and flooded cities out. They called them the Dambusters, and they had flown from an airfield not far from where we lived.

The street boys said, "We bet that was them flying over us the other day. Our pilots are the greatest in the world – nobody can beat them."

My friend and I would play on the trams. One day while playing upstairs on one she saw an open window and climbed through it, pulling herself on to the top of the tram using the rail along the top of it. As she was a foot taller than me she managed it quite easily.

Then she said, "Come on, then, it's your turn."

I said, "I cannot get hold of the rail. I am not tall enough."

She said, "I will pull you up."

She lay across the top, hanging on to the rail, and reached down. I climbed out of the window and, with my feet still on the window ledge, grabbed hold of her hand. She started to try to pull me up, but when I took my feet off the window ledge she could not keep hold of me and let go of my hand. I slid all the way down the side of the tram, which must have been twelve feet high, and I landed on my feet. I could not believe it. I was not hurt – not even a scratch.

She shouted, "Come on, try again. Come back up. I won't let go next time."

But enough was enough for me – once bitten twice shy.

I shouted back, "No, I am not tall enough to reach the railings. I will only fall."

She was mad with me and she climbed back through the window and came back down the stairs. I was swinging on a pole near the open doors, and as she came by me she doubled up her fist and punched me right into the middle of my stomach, leaving me gasping for breath.

Then she ran home, shouting to me as she ran, "I am not your friend ever."

A cleaner came on to the tram to sweep it out and told me to get off home and not to play on the tram again.

Next day we were best of friends. I never said anything to her for punching me, but I thought, 'It's one she owes me.'

Mother would make her own bread. She would mix it in a big bowl – you could always smell the yeast in it – and then put a tea cloth over it and leave it in the hearth overnight to rise. It would rise over the top of the bowl, and then she would put it in tins in the oven. We could not wait for it to bake because then she would cut us a chunk of it. We always called it a doorstep, not a chunk. It was tasty and warm with dripping running on it.

Some people would take their dough to the pawnbroker (we always knew the pawnbroker because he had three brass balls hung up outside his door). He would lend them money on their bowls of dough just for one day.

We would buy a bag of bacon bones from the butcher's. Mother would boil them on the fire. We loved sucking the marrow out of them. Mother would say the marrow was good for us – it would help us to have strong bones.

My young brother had a sit-up-and-beg bike. He went everywhere on it. The tyres were solid, made of hard rubber just like those on babies' prams – the coach-built ones – so it was a bit of a hard ride. My friend and I nicked it one time and took turns on it, going up and down our street. I had just got on it for my second go when I saw him coming after me. I started riding it faster to get away from him, but he caught me. He grabbed hold of the bike and it stopped dead. I fell off it and caught my ankle on the chain as I fell to the floor. It cut right across my ankle and I had to have it stitched, Mother boxed his ears for dragging me off the bike. I felt sorry for him because I knew it was my fault – I should not have nicked his bike; I knew it was his pride and joy. But I was not going to admit it was my fault, for I would have had my ears boxed also for nicking it off him.

My friend and I went window-shopping down Freeman Street now we were going further afield, travelling where there were more shops to look at, and a marketplace. We would walk down one side then the other side looking in the windows. One shop always had a penny-farthing bike on display on a small roof just above the shop. It would fascinate us and we would wonder how anyone could ride on it as one wheel was at least five times bigger than the other one – that is why it was called a penny-farthing. The front wheel was the penny and the back wheel was the farthing because those were the relative sizes, so my brother always told us. My friend and I wanted a sit-up-and-beg bike with a basket on the front.

We travelled right down Freeman Street, walking past Riby Square Hope Street, where we saw three boys on a bomb site. They had some tins and jars lined up and were firing their catapults at them. We stood watching them and admiring what good shots they were. They hit their targets every time, never missing.

They asked us our names and told us theirs. They were three years older than us. They were Robert, George and Roly. They lived in Bedford Street and John Street. We hung around and were stacking their tins up for them to fire at, we so admired them. I held the tins up for Robert as I liked and trusted him – he never missed. I thought he was great. My friend held them up for George. He was small like me and I could see she was not keen on holding them up for him. She was tall like Robert and kept trying to stack his tins up for him, but I was not going to let her – I kept getting them first. After a long time we said we had to go home as we had been out all day. We were not bothered about having our ears clipped for staying out as we had done it many times before and said it was worth it. So we said goodbye to the boys.

Then George said to me, "Give us a kiss, then, before you go." And he kissed me on the cheek and said, "See you again." He then said to Robert, "Go on, then, give her friend a kiss goodbye."

So he kissed her on the cheek.

I was feeling mad at that, but as we were walking away Robert said to me, "Don't I get a kiss off you, Iris?" And he gave me a kiss on the lips and said, "Hope to see you soon."

I was happy as Larry then. I knew he liked me! I was the one he liked, and I liked him as well.

We shouted cheerio and left them, as it was getting dark.

On the way home my friend said to me, "Robert is too tall for you; George is your size, so just leave Robert alone."

I could see by her face she was jealous and angry at me because Robert had kissed me goodbye. I told her I would not leave him alone because he was my boyfriend – it was me he kissed on the lips. He liked me, and when I was old enough I was going to marry him.

She said, "No, you cannot – he is my boyfriend."

Then we started falling out and ended up fighting. And even though she was bigger than me I nearly always won our fights.

As we got down our street she said, "I'm never going to be your friend again, and I really mean it."

And I told her, "Good, because I am not your friend neither."

The days and nights had been full of aeroplanes still dropping bombs on us. While out playing we had to run for shelter from the one enemy plane that would come over now and again and drop a bomb on the railway bridges or the docks. We would call them the bogeymen.

But this year it had been mostly our planes going overhead – Lancasters, Hurricanes, Spitfires and loads and loads of heavy bombers, non-stop. My brother and his street gang told us we were winning the war. We were liberating cities and countries that Hitler had taken and setting them free. They told us Churchill said on the radio that this was our year. We wondered why people were so happy.

My friend and I both went back near the Hope Street 'bombie' hoping to see Robert and his mates. We hung around for a while and they did not come, so we decided to go home. As

61

we were leaving, we saw them. They were heading towards us. When we saw them I felt so happy. We sat talking. They had been trainspotting on the bridge. We started talking about winning the war and one of Robert's friends pointed to the big tower which was in the middle of Grimsby. To us it looked so big it seemed to take a quarter of Grimsby up. It was so high! His friend said that if the enemy dropped a bomb into that tower it would destroy Grimsby, Hull, Cleethorpes and Immingham as it was full of gas. We would all be blown sky-high. We girls were quite frightened about this.

Robert said, "Don't believe a word of it – he likes to scare people." He said that he was always doing it – telling people we would all be blown to bits. He said that if the Jerries did drop a bomb in the tower it would just fizzle out as it was a water tower. We girls were happy about that.

Then they left because they were going to the prisoners' compound to fire their catapults at the prisoners who were imprisoned there. But before they left Robert gave me a kiss and said, "I will see you soon."

George gave my friend a kiss on the cheek and said, "And I will see you soon."

On the way she said to me that she liked George and she was his girlfriend, and I said, "Yes, I like Robert and he is my boyfriend because he sat near me and kissed me goodbye."

Not long after that – about a week later, while coming home from school – we saw Robert and George waiting for us. They said, "We have come to see you two."

So we let our mothers know we were home from school and ran straight back out to them. We went and sat talking on the step bridge about what we would do when we left school. Robert said he would be a fisherman and be skipper on his own boat. George said he would also be a fisherman because his father was one before he was lost at sea. But he also wanted to fish deep-sea like his father had. Robert said his father was a boxer and had won the Lonsdale Belt. He said he would have liked to have had his father's belt when he was old enough, but his mother had sold it. He also said he would have liked to be a boxer, but he could not because he suffered badly from asthma. He said he had to carry an inhaler with him so he could breathe easily, and he showed it to us.

I said, "Never mind. I will look after you when we are older, because I'm going to be a nurse."

But he did not need any looking after from what we had seen of him – he was quite capable of looking after himself.

My friend had no idea what she would be.

We all went to the bomb site and the boys were firing their 'catties' when a plane came over. We never heard any sirens.

We panicked and the boys said, "It's a Jerry – run for it. Bogeyman!"

We ran after them into a bombed-out house – what was left of it – and crouched down watching the plane. It started dropping bombs, and to us girls they looked like pretty toys. They were falling down over the docks, and the noise they made was a bop-bop-bop-bop-bop, then silence. It was so quiet. When they hit the ground there was a loud boom.

The boys were protecting us and we huddled in the bombed-out house, all stooped down, frightened. But I wasn't as frightened as I usually was because I was with Robert and he had his hands on my shoulders.

The plane headed over the docks down the Humber and out into the North Sea.

Robert and George said the plane had dropped doodlebugs – I had heard them being dropped before, but that was the first time I had ever seen them coming down.

I said, "They looked like toys."

Robert said, "Yes, lots of bombs do, but don't ever pick them up."

We told him we knew – our teachers always told us never to pick anything up and they showed us pictures of bombs. We were still shaken up.

They took us home to our doors and they said they would see us again and we kissed them on the cheek.

The very next day we came out of school and Robert was waiting outside. He said George could not come and he asked me if I would go for a walk with him. I said yes. So I let my mother know I was home, then I legged it out smartly before she had time to give me something to do.

He said, "I'll take you to see my granny and grandad. He breeds little chicks."

So we went. They lived in Hamilton Street. We went down a huge alleyway and Robert knocked on their door and his grandad let us in.

Then his grandad said, "Well, our Bobby, who is this pretty young lady?"

He replied, "This is Iris. She lives down King Edward Street. Me and George met her and her friend while trainspotting."

His grandad said, "I bet she is your girlfriend. Come here, our Bobby, I want to whisper something to you."

His grandad was chewing tobacco. Robert went over to him and leant over, putting his ear near his grandad's mouth to listen to what he had to say. With that, his grandad spat his black tobacco into Robert's ear. Robert jumped away from him, wiping the baccy out of his ear and, shaking his head, tried to get it out of his ear hole.

He was shouting at his grandad, calling him a dirty old man, and saying, "You always do that to me."

His grandad was laughing and said, "Well, you always fall for it, don't you, our Bobby? One day you might learn your lesson."

His grandmother came into the room. She was puffing away on a long white clay pipe. She wiped Robert's ear and face, then gave Robert the flannel so he could clean the tobacco off his hands.

She said to him, "Haven't you learnt yet? You know Gramps always catches you with that one, don't you?" Then she said to his grandad, "Don't do that to him again – it's not nice." She said, "Come on, you two, I'll show you the young chicks and eggs."

We followed her outside and walked to a large garden allotment. Robert said that he sometimes went on his grandad's horse and cart with a shovel to collect horse manure off the roads for the vegetable patch, or collected swill from the neighbours to give to the pig they had.

His grandmother opened the door to the shed and in it was an oil heater and shelves full of eggs. She picked one up and said, "Look, they are ready for hatching. We had better close the door to keep the heat in."

She took us to the back of the shed, where there was another heater with a light on and about fifteen little yellow chicks walking around it. There was straw on the floor for them and I thought they were lovely. She let me hold one in my hand.

Then Robert took me to see the big fat pig in the sty. It was grunting. It was a pink pig.

His grandmother gave us a drink of hot cordial and said, "You and your lovely little friend had better make your way home – it's getting late. Don't forget to bring her to see us again some time, our Bobby."

Robert took hold of my hand and walked me home. On the way he asked if I would be his girlfriend and I said yes.

When we got to my house he gave me a kiss and said, "I'll see you next week." He waved to me and smiled.

As I went inside, Mother was waiting for me with her hands on her hips and that look on her face which told me I was dead.

She said, "And just who is that, then, madam?"

I replied, "His name is Robert Brannan and he's my boyfriend. He is a Roman Catholic and we have been to see his grandad's chicks. Robert lives down Bedford Street and is two years older than me."

She said, "Well, my girl, you are not to go with him ever again. You are too young."

I said, "I will go out to play with him when I want to. You won't stop me, so there."

She said, "Oh, won't I? You will do what I tell you to, young lady – and him a Catholic! Do you know they do not believe in divorce or abortion? Whoever he marries will have a dozen children. And besides that, the Catholic Church will not marry you because you are not a Catholic, and you would not be able to christen any children the pair of you have. So do not go near him ever again."

I was angry. I said, "I'm going to see him again and I don't care what you say or do to me. And don't forget you have six children yourself! And you're not a Catholic."

She was so mad at me! She boxed my ears and swung me around by my hair and said, "Get up to bed, and you will be lucky if you ever step foot out of this house again."

I shouted out to her as I went upstairs, crying, "I will get out of this house, you'll see, and when I am old enough I'm going to marry him. I will run away, you will see if I don't."

She said to me, "I'm warning you, madam. I said you were never to see that Bobby Brannan again, or there will be hell to pay."

I went to sleep, crying and hungry. Before I went to school the next day she threatened to punish me within an inch of my life unless I came straight home from school – which I did anyway because Robert wasn't waiting there.

When I returned home after school, she said, "I hope you have not ignored what I said to you. You'd better not see that boy again."

I said, "I have not seen him at all," which was true (I wasn't to see him for ten years after that).

She said, "Good. It's about time you did as I ask you. You're only a child. When you are old enough to have boyfriends I will have no problem with that. But when you do, always remember to keep your hand on your halfpenny."

My best friend and I decided to join the St John Ambulance Brigade. It was only round our corner in Victoria Street, so we went in to see them after school and asked if we could join up.

The leader said, "Well, you are both too young to join – we would not have a uniform to fit you. But I am sure we can find you something you could do to be of help to us. I will have to see your mothers first to see if it will be all right."

Our mothers both said they would be pleased for us to join as it would keep us off the streets and out of trouble. We could go for an hour twice a week after school for as long as we wanted; if we got tired of going we just had to let them know. We felt so grown-up, and we would brag to our street friends that we were members of the St John Ambulance Brigade – we were helping with the war.

On our first night there we were rolling bandages and stacking them in Red Cross boxes. We did this for a couple of weeks, then they let us practise with them at bandaging people up. We were their dummies. We would lie on the floor while they wrapped bandages around our pretend sprains and cuts. We would be covered in bandages and would end up looking like a couple of mummies – even our heads were covered. We would both look at each other and laugh about it.

They taught us how to wrap up broken bones – we would put splints on a leg or an arm and wrap the bandages around it. Sometimes I would practise on my friend, wrapping her up, and then she would take a turn wrapping me up.

They showed us how to bring someone round if they had fainted. We had to sit them up and bend them over slightly, which would make the blood travel around their body again and bring them round. They let us practise with each other at resuscitation. We thought this very funny and never did it right.

We said to our leader that we might be nurses when we were old enough, the only trouble was my friend fainted at the sight of blood. The leader said she might get over it by then, but we did not think so as we had been practising with fake blood while wrapping up fake cuts for months now and she still felt sick and fainted whenever she saw blood. So we both left there.

We followed a group of people one day – they would walk around the parks and the hospital and stand outside singing songs. They told us it was to try and cheer people up and try to make them feel happy, if only for a little while.

We followed them around for a week. But we did not know half of the songs they were singing, so we soon got sick of that.

One day my brother and mother were sitting transfixed near the radio when my brother started jumping up and down, waving his hands in the air, shouting, "We're winning the war! We're winning the war! Rommel's dead, Rommel's dead. Now we are well on our way to reaching Germany. Once we do, Hitler will be finished. We are slowly winning back all that Hitler has taken. This is our year all right." He went running outside, shouting it out to all his street friends.

I told my friend we were winning the war, and she said, "I only hope and pray that is so because I am so sick of everything. I will be glad when we can play outside in peace and quiet, as I heard my mother telling a neighbour the other day that she was so frightened when I went out to play because she never knew if I was going to return home. She said she was worried that I might be killed, but did not want me not to play."

I told her, "All our mothers say that – they do not want to imprison us."

We went conkering with some boys – they climbed the trees and shook them down and we girls gathered them up. We all shared them and the boys challenged us to a conker fight the next day, so we took them on.

That night my brother told me to soak the conkers in vinegar all night to increase my chances in winning, which I did. Then my brother made holes in them and tied string through. Then he wished me good luck.

It was the first time my friend and I had ever played conkers. We met the boys on our front and took it in turns to hit the conkers. Ours smashed when the boys swung at them first time. Theirs took about three hits before smashing. I had one conker that lasted me for two hits. My friend had no hits, so we were well and truly beaten. The boys laughed at us while wallowing in their glory and told us to roast them in the oven next time and then we might get some hits.

Planes started going overhead. We stopped dead and were ready to run for our lives, but one of the boys said, "It's all right, they are ours – they are friendlies. They are doing sorties, and we think and hope that it won't be long before they sort Berlin and Hitler out."

My two older brothers had returned home from being evacuated. The oldest was fifteen, the other one nearly fourteen. The oldest went straight down to the docks and got a job; the second one got a job selling newspapers on the corner of the main street. The papers cost twopence each, but nearly everyone who bought one would give him a threepenny bit and let him keep the penny change. By the end of the week he had earned himself quite a few pennies, so he was happy. And Mother was happy also because apart from having the brothers home, they were also earning money to help her along.

They would walk down our street together on a night, the oldest one singing and yodelling with the other one playing the mouth organ. They sounded great and people would follow them just to listen to them – mostly girls hoping to be their girlfriends.

They would swim in the river with all their mates and dive off the bridge. Of course they would be surrounded by girls, and me and my friend would sit on the side of the bridge watching all the boys. If they asked us if we could swim we would say yes, but we could not. We were only trying to act grown-up, until they said, "OK, we will throw you in." Then we would admit that we couldn't swim.

My father came home from the war. He had been in the army hospital for months, but was now on the road to recovery. When we saw him he still looked sick – he was shaking with the effects of malaria.

The landlord fixed us a proper bath in our house. We were the only ones down our street with a bath fitted. We could turn the taps on and fill it up that way, then pull out the plug and the water ran away.

My friend said, "You are lucky not to have to drag your old tin bath out and fill it up by hand, like we have to in our house."

Mother was very happy. She said that it had got rid of a lot of hard work for all of us. At bath times I felt like a princess lying there soaking away.

The boss in the fish house which was connected to our house gave my father a job and many a time he would come and knock on our door and say, "Can I borrow Iris to open the door of our office as I have left my keys at home," and I would have to climb through a small window which was in our square yard, and which was in the wall of his fish house. Then I would walk along a desk and lift a catch up that opened the door.

He would give me a brass threepenny bit for opening his door for him.

That year Mother had another baby – another redhead, called Sandra. She would sleep in Mother's room in a dresser drawer until she was old enough to come into our bed with us girls.

That night the sirens went and Mother and Father stayed in the house because they did not want to move a newborn baby around just yet. So all of us others spent the night in the shelter on our own. There were only about six other families in there from our street. Bombs were dropping, but the sound they made while falling down was a different sound altogether from anything any of us had heard before. The others in the shelter could not say what they were. We were all trying to think what kind of bombs they could be. They went on all night.

When the all-clear sounded we went back to our house – it was still there. Mother was listening to the radio. An announcer was saying Hitler had some new bombs which were worse than any bombs he had ever had before as they could reach London on their own and did not even need aeroplanes to bring them over. There were called V-2 rockets.

My brother said, "Well, that's all we need! That's us gone! All we can say is it's time we finished him off for good."

It was Christmas 1944 and Mother said we would be entertaining a few friends, including Father's boss. It usually meant half of the police force because we had always had plenty of police friends and often entertained them. With the older boys back home, we had been practising our band together.

We had a huge enclosed backyard. It had four toilets at one end for the fish workers. We put a few tables and chairs out and Father had a barrel of ale and some food. So we put on our Sunday best and waited for our guests to come.

Mother said she hoped things would go all right. We said we hoped there would be no bombs dropping that night.

My oldest brother sang a couple of yodelling songs, while my oldest sister played piano. My second oldest brother played his mouth organ. I played the piano accordion – 'Silent Night' (that was the only tune I had learnt on it up till then). Then we all joined together and sang them a couple of Christmas carols, and afterwards all of us children had something to eat and went to bed, leaving the grown-ups to their ale. Our bedroom window was overlooking the yard, so us girls sat looking through our window, watching. Father was tipsy and showed Mother up because he insisted on singing a song to her, which he often did in front of us to make us laugh. The trouble was it was always the same song. Now he was singing it in front of everyone. The song was 'Seven Years with the Wrong Woman'.

Mother's face was red and she said, "It is nice to know you are your old self again."

We managed to go to sleep after that, and there were no bombs to wake us up.

My oldest brother, who worked down at the dock, wore clogs for his work. All the dock workers wore them. We would hear them 'clogging' along to work early every morning. My father had an iron shoe last which he would mend our shoes on. When my brother's clogs were worn down he would put them on the shoe last and nail horseshoes on them. It made them last longer. All dock workers did the same.

I would take Mother's knives to the knife sharpener who came down our street. He had a pushbike with an iron square tray on the front of it. In the tray was a round stone with a handle in the middle which he would turn and hold the knife against the stone to sharpen it. Mother would put the knife that had to be sharpened in a leather case so I did not cut myself. I liked to take them to be sharpened as I was fascinated by the way the stone wheel spun round.

All our street friends were on our front and two of them were crying. They had lost their fathers at sea. We always tried to cheer each other up. We said we would always sing our song, 'Ally Ally-oh' whenever we lost anyone. Today our friends who had lost their fathers while sailing to fight at El Alamein sat in the middle of the ring. Up to now we had five sat in the middle; today it was seven. So we held hands and walked around them singing our song, but before we sang it we all decided to change our song from 'Ally Ally-oh' to 'El Alamein' because we were dedicating it to our two newly bereaved friends and we thought it more appropriate for them.

EL ALAMEIN

The big ship sails on the deep blue seas
On the deep blue seas, on the deep blue seas.
The big ship sails on the deep blue seas
On the last day of September.
Deep blue seas, deep blue seas,
The big ship sails away.
The big ship sails on the deep blue seas
On the last day of September.
The big ship is sailing to the El Alamein
To the El Alamein, to the El Alamein.
The big ship is sailing to the El Alamein
On the last day of September.
El Alamein, El Alamein,
The big ship sails away.
The big ship is sailing to the El Alamein
On the last day of September.

I lost my father to the deep blue seas,
To the deep blue seas, to the deep blue seas.
I lost my father to the deep blue seas
On the last day of September.

Over the months the number of children sitting in the middle kept growing.

This year the grown-ups had been so happy, including us children. Mother sometimes took us to the park for a picnic after Sunday school. Once there was a Punch and Judy show – it was the first time we had ever seen Punch and Judy. We girls would play ball on the grass and the lads would climb the trees.

One day a couple of boys from our street took my friend and me scrumping. It was our first time at scrumping. They took us down an alley at the side of People's Park, we looked over a wall at the tree we were going to scrump from – they were very small green-looking apples, and we said that they did not look very nice. But the boys said that they were all right. They had scrumped them before and they were crab apples. The boys went over the wall and one climbed up the tree. He sat on a branch shaking the apples down.

He shouted out to us, "Come on, then, pick them up."

But before we climbed over the wall a dog came out of the door of the house. The boy on the ground ran and jumped back over the wall to us. We looked for the other boy, thinking he would have run with him. But no, he was still up the tree, and sat hanging on to the branch with the dog at the bottom of the tree, looking up at him and barking.

We shouted out to him, "Come on, get down."

He said, "I cannot – the dog will get me."

With that a man came out of the house and started walking towards us and to the tree. We all legged it home, leaving the boy behind to face the music. We did not see him until the next day and we asked what had happened. He said the man helped him down from the tree and he let him have fallen apples to take home with him.

So we said, "OK, well, where is our share, then?"

He said, "No, you lot are not having any – you left me to get bitten by that dog, and the man said to leave his apples alone in the future or next time he will fetch the bobbies. And I am never going scrumping with you lot ever again."

We said, "Good, cos we're not going with you ever again either."

He replied, "I don't want you to because you only leave me anyway."

And we went away shouting, "We don't want to play with you – you are not our friend."

The next time we saw the two boys we said we were sorry. Then we were all friends, and one of the boys took us to see planes that his father had made him. They were in his bedroom hanging from the ceiling by string. They were rather good. They looked like they were flying. There were about fifteen in all, and in the middle of them a barrage balloon was hanging. He knew the names of every plane (he also had German planes), Mosquito, Lancaster bomber, Spitfire, Messerschmitt, Hurricane – he named every plane that was there. He said his father was making him a big battleship to put on his dresser.

We told him, "You are very lucky to have a dad that can make you toys like that, and lucky to have a dad at all."

He said he would show us his battleship when it was finished, and we left.

We were now well into 1945 and the skies were full of activity, day and night, non-stop. We had no rest.

One day a policeman said, "Look at that lot of Lancaster bombers going over – they are the ones that carry the big bombs. I would not be surprised if they are going to Germany to drop their bombs."

While out playing we did not know if we had to run or stay. We had to remain alert and ready to run for it, hoping not to have a bomb dropped on us. Whenever a plane came overhead we would look at the street boys, because we knew they would tell us if they were goodies or baddies.

They would tell us girls, "We don't know why you girls are always scaredy-cats. We have the greatest pilots in the world. Our pilots can shoot a dozen enemy planes down in one go and our gunships are ace and our Allies are so brave. We have already taken back nearly all that Hitler has taken and it won't be long now before everybody will be free."

The boys always made us girls feel good. But we would still worry – because of the planes droning over our heads we could not help wondering if this was to be our last play day. But how relieved we were when that voice would shout out, "It's OK, they're ours – they are friendlies."

We had to go into church every day for morning service at St Barnabas, which was on the way to school. We could not get out of it as Mother would make sure we went inside to thank the Lord for another day. Mother's family were very religious – everything was church and Sunday school. Our Sunday school was the Baptist tabernacle down Victoria Street.

Every time I came home from school Mother would say to me, "Have you seen anything of that Bobby Brannan, your so-called boyfriend? Has he been hanging outside your school for you?"

I would say, "No, I have not seen him."

She would reply, "Good job! Let us hope it stays that way, because he will have forgotten all about you by the time you grow up. He will have married someone else, and so will you."

I told her, "No, I will never marry anyone else but him. He will be my husband, I know he will."

And this would be true, ten years later.

The radio never stopped talking about the war, and my mother would say to us, "That's another country our brave boys and Allies have liberated."

My father said, "Yes, but everybody is concerned about the

German submarines because they are blowing up lots of our merchant ships."

But my brother told us not to worry, and the Yanks would soon sort them out. He said they would soon destroy the German submarines, and later they did just that.

I knew I would not like to fight a war while in a submarine, because one day our teacher took us to see one in the docks. We went inside one to look around. When I first saw it I looked at it and went all cold inside and frightened. It was a long, black, horrible round piece of steel. Inside wasn't much better. As we passed through round doors of steel from room to room, moving along it, I felt no warmth, just coldness. Our teacher was explaining what each room was for, but I was not taking anything in; I wasn't listening to a word he was saying. And I was happy when we got out of it. I thought to myself, 'I feel sorry for anyone, friend or foe, who has to sail in one of them.' To me was a cold iron coffin.

We all got stuck in one day to help Mother with two kitbags full of fishermen's washing as she had to get it all washed and dried for the next two days. She said if we helped her we would get a silver sixpence to share. We did not need to be asked twice.

My oldest sister boiled the long johns in the wash-house boiler while I bashed the fishermen's jumpers about in the dolly tub with a dolly. Then we rinsed them in the tub under the wringer and put them through it, then pegged them on the line. Mother was well pleased, and we got our silver tanner and shared it between us. Those two fishermen never came home. They got lost at sea. Mother said their trawler had been sunk.

My friend and I would cut models out of magazines then stick them on cardboard, cut round them, then cut fancy dresses out of the magazines, making sure to cut tags on them so we could wrap the tags round our models, dressing them with different cut-outs.

One night in my friend's house we were sat playing records

when her brother came into the room. He bent down to light the fire, which had already been made up. He had just lit the paper in the grate when out shot a mouse, and it ran straight up his trouser leg. My friend and I jumped on top of the table. We both stood there screaming and holding our skirts tightly round our bent knees. Her brother had gone deathly white and was thrashing around on his legs with his hands. He was jumping up and down and running around in circles. He stopped dead and dragged off his trousers, running outside with them, throwing them on the ground and stamping on them. He killed the mouse and put his trousers back on.

We both came down off the table and were laughing hysterically.

He said to us, "I don't see what is so funny myself!"

We called him mousy pants and told all his friends, who also would call him mousy pants and ask him if he still had a Wee Willie Winkie.

Father said to my oldest sister and my youngest brother, "Go get me some tab ends from out the gutters as I haven't got a smoke for work tomorrow."

They often went 'tab-ending' for him. I followed them. We found a few, then my brother said he knew where we could find loads. He took us into the trolleybus depot, where the trolleybuses were cleaned for the next day. They threw all the rubbish into big bins, so we scavenged in them and got loads. We took them home and Father undid them on to a newspaper and had a load of baccy for work. He was well pleased.

Our friends knew that sometimes we had to go tab-ending because they had seen us picking them up out of the gutters, and if we fell out with them they would say to us, "You have to go tab-ending out the gutters." And would chant to us; "Dog-enders, tab-ending."

I would feel ashamed and tell Mother what they would call us.

She would say, "You have nothing to be ashamed of – it is them who should be ashamed for mocking you. Never mind, and while they are calling after you they were leaving some other child alone. One day they will realise that we are going through a war and hard times. We live in a world where we cannot have everything we need, so we have to make the best of it."

We called on Lizzie. We had not been to see her for ages. It was cold outside and she made us a hot cup of cocoa. We sat round her fire talking – she always told us stories about when she was a young lady. She said she used to live abroad and she was one of Al Capone's girlfriends and he would buy her pearls and jewels. She said she loved him as he was so kind to her, but he had to go to jail, so she came to live in Grimsby and married a young soldier. But he got killed in the First World War and she never had any children and would never marry again.

When I got home I asked my mother who Al Capone was because old Lizzie had said he was her boyfriend and a very famous person. She told me not to believe what old Lizzie said as she was always spinning yarns.

My two older brothers were now at home, and the eldest one wanted a bedroom of his own. So one of my sisters (the one eight months younger than me) and I had to sleep in a bed in Mother's room until we had things sorted out. Our new baby was staying with my mother's sister for a while. Mother's room was the only room in the house that had a gas heater in it. One night Mother, my sister and I had gone to bed for the night. It was a bit cold and I remember Mother telling me to switch the heater on. I reached out and turned it on, and I don't remember any more until I woke up in hospital. I had been unconscious and Mother and my sister were in a hospital bed next to me.

Mother said, "It's about time you woke up," and she shouted to a nurse.

The nurse came to me and said, "We have been waiting for you to open your eyes. You have been gassed. You are the last to wake up. Your mother and sister have been awake for days."

Mother then told me what happened. The heater had not lit when I turned it on and the gas escaped, gassing us three.

Our two older brothers had been sat downstairs telling ghost stories and one of them said, "Can you smell gas?"

He got up and walked to the bottom of the stairs, where it smelt so strong. They shot upstairs and found us all unconscious from the gas. They turned it off and dragged us out of the house into the street and we went to the hospital.

I had my head nearest the heater – that's why they think I took the longest to come round. Mother, my sister and I had a good cry and we thanked our brothers for saving our lives.

It was a terrible accident. It took me years to get over the smell of gas. Every time I smelt oil or petrol I would be violently sick.

My brother said, "Isn't it ironic – we live in fear of Hitler gassing us, and my mother and sisters were gassed with our own gas."

We had a good year for not being bombed. Although the skies were full of planes going and coming, they were ours. We were getting the odd bogeyman over our town. My brothers said it was because we were hitting them where it counted. They were getting more than they could give us and soon we would be reaching Berlin, so now we would see how the Germans could take it on their own doorstep.

My oldest sister took me with her to the ice-skating rink. I had never been on ice skates before. I was an excellent skater on my roller skates and I was a bit concerned about it, but she told me that roller skates were harder to skate on than ice skates, so I should do all right. Then I was excited and could not wait to go. We arrived and went inside. It was full of airmen and soldiers skating around the rink. We went and tried on the skates. I had a nice pair of white ones. I went on the rink with my sister holding my hand. It was not long before I got the hang of it and started going round on my own, thinking to myself, 'She is right, this is a lot easier than my roller skates.'

I started doing twirls and spins, which I always did on my roller skates. I found it so much easier and loved it on the ice. I got so carried away with myself I was gliding around with one leg up in the air like a ballet dancer in Swan Lake – that is what I felt like. I was really showing off. Suddenly I noticed that nearly all the airmen and the army men had stopped skating and were watching me and my performance. I felt embarrassed, went quite red and skated off to where my sister was. Then they all clapped me, shouting, "Bravo."

My sister and I did a few more laps round then went home.

She told my mother how good I was on the ice.

Mother said, "Oh, she would. She has always been a clever little show-off. One day will come her downfall."

One of my brothers told us girls about one of the boys who had worked with him on the farm he was evacuated to. They were driving a tractor down the field when the boy decided to sit on the front of it for a ride. The field was full of stones and the tractor hit a big one and the boy fell off. He fell to the ground and one of the big back wheels of the tractor ran over his legs. There were other workers in the field watching them and saw the tractor run over him. They gasped in horror at it, and they ran to him to see if they could help him in any way, all thinking the worst. He got up off the ground laughing. He was lucky – the wheel had pushed him under the soft muddy soil. The only thing that was wrong with him was the tractor had ripped the backside of his trousers out and all his bum was showing, so they got him a cloth potato sack, cut holes in the bottom of it for his legs and tied it round his waist with string. He worked all day in the potato sack.

The same boy another time had been cleaning out the horse stables and was patting a horse on its head. Then he started showing off, saying to the horse, "Give me a kiss." It gave him a kiss all right – it bit him on his lips, taking a lump out of them and scarring him for life.

I was playing 'faggies' when Mother came outside with my baby sister. She strapped her in her high chair on our doorstep and said for us to keep an eye on her while she got her work done. We carried on playing with the fag cards, but suddenly sirens started going off. Mother came running out. She undid the baby straps, telling us to run for shelter. She took the baby out of the high chair, but she got the straps caught on herself and the baby fell to the floor. Mother tried to stop her fall and she managed to catch her, but the baby still caught her head on the floor. Our baby sister started crying.

Mother felt all over her head and said, "At least she is not bleeding – I think she's just bruised." She ran into the house with her, telling us to get to the shelter.

Before we got the chance, two planes were flying overhead and we stood gaping at them.

My brother said, "One is a Jerry and the other one is ours. Look, they are having a dogfight."

We stood there looking at them. We were transfixed. One was going really fast in front of the other one, which was right behind him, following him. They were both zigzagging in a line in the sky, and the one in front shot up into the sky in a straight line with the other one following on his tail. The one in front went silent as if he had turned his engine off, then his plane began falling out of the sky, spinning round in circles. After about four circles his engine came back to life as if it had been turned on. It made a big swoop round in the air with the other one still on its tail and shot straight up into the sky in a straight line then dropped right down again. My brother said that it was trying to dive-bomb the plane that was keeping on its tail. Then we saw a trail of fire coming from the second plane. My brother said that one was ours, but it had just fired at the Jerry plane, which started falling down out of the sky with a trail of blackish smoke behind it. It went down over North Cotes, falling out of sight. Our plane started flying towards Lincoln, and as it flew off it tipped its wings a couple of times before flying out of sight.

My brother said, "Did you see that? He tipped his wings. Well, that means triumph – that means victory!"

The sirens went for the all-clear and we went inside our house.

Mother was holding our baby sister over the sink, putting cold water on her head. She was very upset. The baby's head was all swollen – it felt and looked like a sponge. The baby was sobbing. Mother said she would have to take her to the hospital and I went with her. They gave her an X-ray and said she was all right. Mother had to take her back there every week for her to have her head massaged. The doctor who did this massage had no fingers – only stumps on both hands, which he would rub all over the baby's head. Mother told me his hands had special powers in them – they were healing powers. After a month the baby's head was better – the swelling had all gone. We had our baby sister all fit and well.

We told Father about the two planes dogfighting over Grimsby, and he said he and the fish workers had seen them through the works window.

My friend and I wanted to join the Brownies, like some of our street friends. So we went to ask if we could join. The lady said we could have a trial, and if we liked it and wanted to stay we could buy the uniform.

That Sunday all of us Brownies met in a room at our Baptist tabernacle. Mother said she would buy me the Brownie outfit if I stayed in it, but she did not think I would stick at it for long anyway. She said my friend and I never did stick at things.

The leader met us at the tabernacle. She had a horse and cart. We all climbed on it as we were going out into the countryside. There were ten of us children. We travelled into a big field and all climbed out of the cart. The leader said, "Go in pairs and collect twigs and stumps of wood to make a fire. Stay together and bring it all back here to make one fire."

So I went with my friend and the others as we collected our twigs from a small wood alongside the field. We all took them back to the field, where our leader was waiting, and we piled them all together. Then our leader lit the fire. She told us on our next assignment she would be showing us how to light the fire without a match.

Then we took it in turns to fry an egg on the fire. We had not had an egg before. We had always had powdered eggs at home.

The leader said the farmer's wife had given us the eggs.

When it was my turn she gave me the pan, and I cracked my egg in it and held it over the fire. What a mess it was, black with smoke, but I ate it. My friend's was the same as mine, and even though we felt sick at the sight of it we did not want the leader to think we could not be a Brownie like the others, so we ate it and felt proud of ourselves because we had done the same as them.

The horse and cart came and took us to the farmhouse. We went inside and we sat on a big rug on the floor near a huge fire. The farmer's wife gave us all a drink of milk, then she played the piano for us and asked if any of us could sing. I said I could as I was in my school choir. I thought to myself, 'I have opened my mouth again without thinking.' My friend always said I had a big mouth.

She said, "OK, you can sing for us!"

So I got up and sang, and the farmer's wife played the piano to my song, which was 'All Things Bright and Beautiful'.

Afterwards we had to thank the farmer and his wife for the use of his field. The farmer told our leader we can go any time in his field for our Brownie days out. We went back home on the horse and cart to our Brownie hut. The leader said me and my friend had passed our trial – we were fully fledged Brownies. My mother was not right this time – saying my friend and I would not stay long – because we got our Brownie uniforms and we were Brownies for five years.

One day I was lying in bed making castles out of the patches on the ceiling when I heard screaming outside. I got out of bed and went to look out of the window. My sister followed me. There was an army man and woman outside our house shouting at each other and fighting.

He knocked her to the ground, banging her head up and down on the pavement, then got up and was kicking her, shouting, "You are not bringing that Yank's baby in our house. I will kill you first."

We both started screaming for Mother. She came running into our bedroom.

My sister and I were crying, "Mother, that man is kicking that lady on the floor. He is going to kill her!"

She looked out of the window, then closed the curtains, saying, "Get back in bed the pair of you. What have I told you about opening the curtains? You will get me into trouble one of these days. Don't ever let me catch you opening them again, or else I will let your father deal with the pair of you."

We both said, "But, Mother, that man and woman are fighting."

She said, "And that is none of your business and certainly none of mine. So don't ever forget that. Now, don't let me hear a word from either of you again."

When I called for my friend for school the next day the neighbours were all stood talking about what happened, and we stood earwigging. They were saying someone had told the husband that, while he was away fighting, his wife had been going out with an American airman. The husband had been taken away in a Black Maria and she had been taken to hospital and had lost her baby. Then my friend's mother said we should stop earwigging and get off to school before we got our ears boxed.

When we got to school we always had to line up in front of our desk for our teacher's inspection. He would go down the line to check if our hands and shoes were clean. If they were dirty we would get the cane. He was halfway down the line with his inspection when I looked down at my feet. There were scuff marks on my white sandshoes.

I thought, 'Oh no, that's me for the cane.'

I had had the cane quite a few times now and I, like the others, would hold out my hand and take the whack without showing any pain. But nevertheless it still hurt somewhat. I saw the teacher getting nearer. I panicked, looked behind me and spotted the teacher's chalk on the board. Then I had a brainwave. I picked the chalk up off the backboard and rubbed it all over my sandshoes, then put the chalk in my pocket as I never had time to put it back on his board because he was right near me by now. He looked at me. It worked!

He said, "OK, go sit at your desk."

I kept his chalk for future emergencies.

My friend said to me, "I saw you, you crafty devil, with the teacher's chalk. I am going to keep some chalk in my pockets also for my sandshoes because chalk is better than whitewash – your shoes look much cleaner than mine."

One day in 1945 Mother and Father got all of us children together. I thought to myself, 'Oh no! What has happened now? They only gather us all together when something bad is happening.'

But this time they were both smiling. They said to us, "We have won the war, thank God. Thank the Lord. The war has ended – we are free and we are alive."

Father said there were still a few places that we had to clear up yet, but we had won. Hitler was dead.

My brother said, "Have we dropped a bomb on him, then?"

Father said, "No, Hitler shot himself. He committed suicide. It is finished. The radio told us Winston Churchill is telling all the people that the war is ending. War is over. We have won. And he is doing a victory V sign with both hands."

So us children were doing it with both hands and laughing and shouting, "It's VE day – war is over."

The radio told us the Royal family were out on the balcony of Buckingham Palace, which was surrounded with great crowds of people, and the King was saying how great the people were. All of us children went outside, where crowds were gathering in the street. Our neighbours were putting flags across the street from window to window. We were laughing because some of them had hung big bloomers across the street. People were cheering and dancing. We had to make sure we did not get crushed because the roads and pavements were so full of people. We had never seen so many together in our lives.

My older brother said not to go into the square near the town hall because it was even worse – full of army, air force and navy servicemen, and people were climbing up lamp posts and leaning out of windows, listening to the mayor giving a speech from the balcony of the town hall.

We had to go back inside our house and just look out of our windows because otherwise we would have been crushed. People were singing and dancing in the streets – parties and cheering went on for days.

At night I did not put my head under the covers, but we could not sleep because of all the singing and cheering going on.

Months later the radio told us that an atomic bomb had been dropped on Japan – Hiroshima. We were still clearing up loose ends, so Father would tell us. Then Japan surrendered – everyone called it VJ day.

My friends and I could play outside together without worrying about bombs dropping on our heads. We would always have a house to live in. We would not be coming out of our shelters and finding our houses gone – blown up.

We could play games right through to the end without having to bolt for cover without fearing for our lives.

The sirens were silent. All we heard all night were the fishing boats, all sounding their foghorns, and the church bells ringing out with happiness.

No more blackouts, no more blackness. We could have our lights on all night if we wanted to. We did not have to come home from school in the dark, having to feel our way along by touching the walls.

Mother and Father were happy and sad; Mother had lost two of her brothers, who were pilots, and Father had three brothers missing in action, missing at sea. They were sailors.

My father came from Jarrow – he was a Geordie. He had seven brothers; now there were only five.

Every time we earwigged the subject was always who was killed, or who was missing. All so young and brave!

When we met our street friends we had to comfort each other. We decided to sing our El Alamein song, but there were so many of us to sit in the middle because of loss of loved ones and friends that we decided no one would sit in the middle; we all walked round and sang our original song, 'Ally Ally-oh', holding hands.

Months later we lost half of our street friends. They emigrated to Australia, New Zealand and Canada.

What is this life that we did share?
Running around, but full of fear,
Our nerves were all shattered,
Some of us in mourning,
Which of us to wake in the morning?
Putting on a brave face
While coming and going,
Smiling and laughing,
But most of us knowing,
Terrified, frightened,
Struck dumb with emotion,
That when we returned home
Whose hearts will be broken?
Fighting and killing,
Some of us sinning,
Some of us losing,
Some of us winning,
Hearts full of love.
So who can we turn to?
So who can we tell?
One thing for certain:
We had six years of hell.
Now war has ended
We can all start anew,
Our lives awaiting
For us to go to.

THANK YOU, LORD

Thank You for the world so sweet,
Thank You for the food we eat,
Thank You for our friends, our play,
Thank You, Lord, for another day.

Amen.

PART TWO

MY LIFE AFTER THE WAR

My friend or my enemy,
My husband, my life,
My children, my joy,
My pain, my strife.

Prologue

It was playtime and my best friend and I were playing skipping when a girl asked us, "Can I play with you?"

I was just going to say, "You can play if you like."

But before I could say one word my friend said, "No, you cannot, so clear off and don't ask us again!"

With that the girl grabbed my friend by her hair, threw her on the ground, jumped on her and started smacking her in the face. I grabbed the girl off her and gave her a good kicking.

She ran off, shouting out, "You two are for it now. Just you wait till my friends get hold of you!"

Then the bell rang and we went to our classrooms.

At home time there were six of them waiting. They were bigger than us – in their last year. We ran across to the Boulevard toilets and locked ourselves in. They were banging on the door for a while, then they told my friend if she opened the door they would let her go, they would not hit her. I could not believe it – she opened the door. They let her go and gave me a good kicking. My friend walked home with them, telling them she would be their friend. She had betrayed me. I had been her friend for nine years, and we had been through the war together, through thick and thin. Now she had cast me aside, thrown me to this gang after I had protected her from that girl.

I told myself I would never be her friend again. Now she was my enemy.

In the morning she called for me, everything forgotten. I walked to school holding hands with my friend.

School assembly song –

JERUSALEM

And did those feet in ancient time
Walk upon England's mountains green?
And was the holy Lamb of God
On England's pleasant pastures seen?

And did the Countenance Divine
Shine forth upon our clouded hills?
And was Jerusalem builded here
Among these dark Satanic mills?

Bring me my bow of burning gold!
Bring me my arrows of desire!
Bring me my spear! O clouds, unfold!
Bring me my chariot of fire!

I will not cease from mental fight,
Nor shall my sword sleep in my hand,
Till we have built Jerusalem
In England's green and pleasant land.

Starting School, 1949

My mother had bought me my first school uniform, now I was eleven years old starting big school. I loved it. I was now grown-up. The uniform consisted of a black pleated gymslip ('jolly hockey sticks' style), a striped tie and sash belt that all of us girls would leave dangling down so it nearly touched the floor, a black blazer and beret, both with the school badge on the front, and a brown leather satchel.

My best friend had the same as me because we were both going to the same school again. This was Armstrong Secondary Modern Girls' School. If anyone asked us what school we went to we always said, "Armo."

Our school was separated from the boys' by a gate in both playgrounds. And every playtime the gate would come flying open and a boy would come flying into our playground, having been thrown through the air by the other boys. Then the gate would close and they would lock it so the boy could not get back into his own playground. To do so he had to pass by all of us girls and go round our part of the school and right round the front of the school to reach his own school. They also would take one of his shoes and throw it on the high roof. We girls would be staring at him and laughing because his face would be bright red and he would be half walking, half running with his head down, so embarrassed, trying to get out of there as quickly as he could and get back to his home ground.

My friend and I were lucky again – we were in the same class. We had to catch a tram to school because it was a good distance from our homes. It was right over the marsh. But most times we would spend our one-penny tram fare and walk. Shanks's pony, as Mother would call it.

"Use your legs that the good Lord gave you." She always said that to us if she did not have the tram fare for us.

Sometimes we had no intention of walking. We would run behind the horse and carts that carried wood to the woodyards. The man driving the cart always slowed down until we got on to the planks of wood, then he would speed up again. Once we reached school he would slow down so we could jump off.

We soon made many friends. We found out some of them had a lot of bad ways, but if we wanted to be in their gang we had to copy them. One morning we followed them and, as we reached the Boulevard – which was only one corner away from our school – they all ran inside and went up on a swing. We joined them because we wanted to be their friends.

We had a few swings and then said, "We had better go now or we will be late for school."

They told us, "If you want to hang around with us, just shut up and do what we do. We are not going into school – we are twagging today." ('Twagging' is slang for playing truant.)

So we carried on swinging away, enjoying it. Some children who were in our class had seen us and told our teacher that we were playing on the Boulevard, and the next thing we knew we looked down and there stood the headmistress and our teacher looking up at us. They had walked across from our school to take us back. There were seven of us on the swings, swinging away merrily until we spotted them.

The head said to us, "You may as well stop that swing and come down this instant, the lot of you. We know you intended playing truant, but now you have been caught out. I suggest you all come down from there. Come to school with us and accept your punishment."

Two of our so-called new friends stopped swinging and joined them.

We carried on swinging away defiantly until our teacher said, "You will have to come down sometime today. We can wait all day if we need to. It will be worse for you!"

We knew they were right, so we all stopped swinging and got down. They frogmarched us to school and into the headmistress's study. We had to stand in line facing them while they decided what punishment to dish out to us. In the end we had to report to the head's study each morning before class to prove we had arrived at school for a full week. We would be caned two mornings running in front of our classmates, letting them know that it was for playing truant. We also had to write fifty lines of 'I must not play truant from school.'

That was not the first time we had been in trouble for hanging around with them. Another time on the way to school they said, "Come on, we will show you two how to have fun while going to school."

We lagged behind them. The street on the way to school was full of shops selling different goods. They went into the first shop – it sold wallpaper. They picked up rolls of wallpaper and hurled them all over the shop floor, then they legged it outside and ran into the next shop, laughing along the way. They went inside and then threw potatoes and onions about the shop, and even threw some at the shopkeeper behind the counter, then ran back outside.

We did not copy them – we wanted nothing to do with that. We felt ashamed. We liked having fun, but not that kind. We had been brought up to respect people; we were still churchgoers and still went to Sunday school. We did not think that was funny.

We stayed behind when the gang ran away for the next so-called fun. We knew this shopkeeper – we had been to his shop when we were at infant school in the war. He would tell us stories about when he was a young lad in the First World War. We told him how sorry we were for what the gang had done and we helped him pick up his goods and put them back on display. We told him we thought the gang's pranks were unacceptable and we would be telling our headmistress. He said that he hoped we would pop in now and again like we used to. He had remembered us visiting him during the Second World War.

When we got to school we reported them like we said we would, and we had to go round to the boys' school to pick the boys out, and round our school to pick the girls out. The headmistress said we had done the right thing because that gang of girls and boys had done the same thing many a time on the way to school and had even injured one of the shopkeepers. She told us they would be punished for it and she was happy that we had the sense not to join in.

The next day after school, they were waiting for us. There

were five of them, three girls from our school and two boys from the boys' school.

"Telltale tits, your mother's got nits and your father walks with a walking stick," they chanted at us, then they approached us to hit us.

I went for the ringleader, who was the gobbiest of them – and a boy, I might add. My brother always said if a gang ever went for me I should always go straight for the gobby one – the leader – so I did. I whacked him one right in his face, then I kicked him where it hurt. My friend was dragging a girl along the floor by her hair. They had soon had enough and all ran away, calling us names as they legged it.

My oldest sister and my brother went to the same school as us. My sister was nearly ready for leaving school – she was in her last year. She knew that gang and she warned them that if they touched us again they would have her gang to deal with. So they kept their distance from us when we saw them at home time, but they still chanted after us.

My last name was Usher, so they chanted after us from afar:

'Usher, the pusher the pram,
She made a jar of jam.
She chased me round the market clock
And dropped her jar of jam.'

We would shout after them, "If we catch hold of you we will wipe the floor with the lot of you, just wait and see!"

They always chanted at us from a long way behind us. They were frightened to come anywhere near us because they knew my sister's gang would deal with them. Not that we needed them to fight our battles for us anyway, as we always gave a sight more than we received. There were not many who dared to stand up to us – they always ran away

Me and my friend fell out over our art teacher. We thought he looked like a film star, we thought him so handsome and good-looking. We were in love. We would argue over which of us

93

we thought he would take more notice of. We hated each other because she thought he liked her best and I thought he liked me best. We got some lipstick so we could get dolled up to see who he liked the best. When it came to art lessons we both lathered it on our lips. We walked into the room, smiling at him, with a stupid sway of our hips.

He looked at the pair of us and said, "You two madams come with me; the rest of you carry on with your work till I get back."

Then he marched us both to the headmistress. He spoke to her in another room.

After a while they both returned and said to us, "Do you two know the rules of this school? Rule one, you cannot wear lipstick. Rule two, you cannot eat on the way to school. Rule three, these rules must not be broken. The pair of you will write them down fifty times at playtime and you will be caned in front of your class so they can learn from it also!"

He took us back and caned us in front of our class, saying, "You two have been caned for wearing lipstick in school and breaking school rules." Then he took us to the toilets and said, "Don't come back into class until you have washed your dirty faces."

So on the way home we were the best of friends and we both agreed that our art teacher was an ugly, horrible old man and we did not like him one bit because he had split on us and told us we had dirty faces.

We would often take a shortcut to school through an alleyway as it would cut a full street off our journey. Going through it one morning there was a man stood in the bend of it. As we got near him he opened his coat and exposed himself to us. We looked up and were gobsmacked and scared. We had never seen the like of that before in all our lives, for we thought it looked like a huge bargepole. But what a huge bargepole looked like we had no idea. We had heard it mentioned before, though, by a neighbour about her daughter's boyfriend. She had said he was built like a big brick shite house and her daughter would never leave him because he had a huge bargepole. We did not find out anything else because they told us to clear off and stop earwigging or else our ears would fall off.

Me and my friend stood there wondering what to do. We were struck dumb with fright. Then I grabbed hold of her hand and we both ran like the clappers out of there. We did not run his way, though – we did a U-turn and ran out the way we had gone in. We had no intention of going by him, no thank you. When we had calmed down somewhat we then carried on to school, but we did not take any more shortcuts; we stayed on the main route all the way there and decided to tell our headmistress about it. We told her and we had to stay in her study till a policeman came to talk to us. We told him everything and he took us home. On the way we had to show him the alleyway. He explained to our mothers and told them that they would catch him. We had the rest of the day off school. Mother made sure we went to school on the tram and warned us not to take any more shortcuts down alleyways in the future.

About a week later Mother told us they had caught the horrid man and he would be punished, and she said if we ever saw anything like that again we must always tell someone straight away.

We liked doing PE at this school because we would be taken out of school to do it on the Boulevard. We played tennis, hockey and netball.

One day we were playing tennis – there were four of us on our court playing doubles. None of us had played it before – we were all learning. We paired up. I swung my racket in the air to whack the ball, and I whacked it all right, but as my racket came back down it landed right in the face of my partner, who was playing alongside me. She fell to the ground, holding her face and screaming. Her nose was teeming with blood. The teacher tried to stop the bleeding, but had to take her to hospital to have her checked over. The hospital was right alongside the Boulevard. A prefect had to take us all back to school and explain to our headmistress what had happened. We carried on with our lessons. Later, before home time, we were told the girl had a broken nose and nobody was to blame as it was an accident.

I had to take a bag of Mother's washing to the bag wash, not far from our street. It was near Riby Square. I called for my friend and she went with me. I slung the washing over my shoulder – it was all inside a white pillowcase. We washed and dried it and started back home.

Then my friend had a brainwave. She said, "Come on, I know a shortcut back home." And she started walking down a passageway.

I was warned by my mother never to go down alleyways again as it was dangerous, but what did I do? I started following her. So we walked and we walked and we walked. It was never-ending. I kept asking her, "Are we nearly there yet or what?"

She said, "Yes, come on, it's not far now; we are nearly there."

The washing was getting heavier and heavier. We eventually came out the other side. I could have killed her when I found out where we were. If I had not been carrying the washing and was not knackered I would have done so. We had ended up halfway to Cleethorpes. I was flaming mad at her. It was getting dark.

I told her, "I've just about had enough of you and your shortcuts. Just keep them to yourself in future."

I started back home on the main road. It would be longer, but at least we would not get lost again. And I was determined that would be the last alleyway I would ever go down.

I was so tired by now and she would not take a turn in carrying the washing, my friend, my enemy.

We passed a woman holding a young boy's hand. The boy shouted out and pointed at me. "Look, Mummy, there is Father Christmas and he has a sack of toys."

People passing by looked and laughed and my sinful friend was also laughing.

She kept taking the mickey, saying, "Come on, Santa, your mother's waiting for her sack of toys."

I said, "I don't think you are funny in the least and it is all your fault in the first place. Stuff your shortcuts and stuff them where the sun don't shine."

She said, "Now now, I was only trying to help you get home quicker."

I said, "You can help someone else. Leave me out in future. I hate you! You are an enemy to me – you are not a good friend."

Was I glad when I finally reached home!

When I got in, Mother said, "You two have been a long time. What happened? Did you get lost or something?"

She did not know how near the truth she was.

I just shrugged my shoulders and said, "Yeah, something like that!"

My friend said, "Well, I'll be getting home, then. I'll see you tomorrow."

I said to her, "Are you sure you would not like me to show you a shortcut home?" She only lived six houses away.

She said, "No, you're all right, I think I can find my own way, thank you very much!"

She left, but not before I stared a few daggers her way.

Coming home from school one day, as we reached our street we could see that it was full of our neighbours. They were watching a fight. I could not believe it – it was my oldest brother and his best friend. They were really laying into each other. We stood watching them with the rest of the crowd. There were two policemen trying to break it up, but every time they tried they got knocked back out of the way. They were throwing punches at one another and the punches would send them flying across the road. So one policeman brought my mother out, and she told my brother to stop fighting and got in between the two of them. They did not want to hurt her, so they stopped. They and the policemen went into our house to sort it out.

They had been fighting over a girl who had been going out with both of them, telling each she was their girlfriend. They both agreed to dump her – which they did. The police warned them to keep the peace.

One of my mother's brothers would visit us sometimes, and me and my friend would always con him. As he was leaving I would say, "Uncle Johnny, have you got a penny for us so we can buy some peanut butter?"

He would always give us a penny each. We had been conning him for years – it always worked.

When we were fourteen years old we would go to the roller-skating rink in Wonderland, Cleethorpes. After skating we would stroll along the beach near the pier. We strolled along the pier not long after a great storm had hit Cleethorpes hard. It had washed loads of games machines into the sea and loads of sideshows, slot machines and even some of the pier, and further down it washed some of the caravan park away with some of the caravans being washed out to sea. It was carnage.

This day as we strolled along the beach we spotted loads of pennies in the sand. The tide had gone out. We took our roller skates out of our bags and started filling our bags with pennies. After a while, when we could not find any more, we took them home to my house and counted them. Our bags were full and heavy – we had at least 400 pennies. When we finished counting we had a pound each, which was a week's pay for most people. I shared mine out: I gave my mother ten shillings and bought myself some new clothes. Ten shillings I spent myself, giving my brothers and sisters a share of my ten. My friend shared hers with her family.

After skating the following week we went back to the same place, hoping to find more. We waited for the tide to go out, and we walked up and down that beach, but we did not find one penny. We tried a couple more times after that, but all we found were three halfpennies.

I was beginning to hate my father – he had changed since coming home from the war. He was always hitting my mother. He would give her the rent money, then he would ask for it back and when she would not give it to him he would hit her. He had been hitting her for quite a number of years now.

One day he was asking her for money and he went to grab

her. She ran upstairs to get away from him, but he ran after her and I ran behind them. He had pinned her up against the wall with the big iron bed, squashing her with it. I was screaming at him to leave her alone. Then my older sister came running into the room. She had just come home from work, where she was training to be a nurse. She started lashing out at him to leave our mother alone. He ran out of the house, but kept threatening my mother as he ran. My two older brothers were home now (they had been doing their national service). One had been in Korea and the other had been in the Malayan jungle. They had warned him about hitting her before when they were fifteen and sixteen years old. They would put their mitts up to him, but he would just laugh at them and box their ears.

They would say to him, "When we are older and stronger we will throw you out." And now they were strong young men.

As soon as they came home we children told them that Father had squashed Mother with the bed.

When my father came back into our house they gave him a good hiding. My father had a big lump on his head.

He packed his bags and left, with my brothers shouting after him, "Don't ever set foot in this house again or you will get more of that treatment."

All of us children were so happy to see him go because every time he hit Mother we could not help her. We had to just watch it, and I had hated him for it for years. At long last we would not have to see him hitting our mother again.

Over the years of him hitting her I would look at my friend's father, the way he was so loving and kind to his wife and children, and I would think to myself, 'I wish I had a nice father, like him.' Instead I had a nasty, evil father I hated more each day. But now I could not be happier. At last he was gone and I don't think he would dare to come back while my brothers were home. We were so proud of them.

Starting Work

My friend and I were now fifteen and had just left school. We had just got our first job together. My oldest sister was a nurse now, working at the Springfield Hospital in the TB ward. My friend and I started working at Scribbs and Kemps Biscuit Factory, Great Coates. We had to catch a train from Grimsby Town Station to get there. There were about fifteen of us from Grimsby working there, so we would all sit in the same carriage for a chinwag and a laugh.

One night on the way home after work all of us girls were laughing and joking together when a young man came into our carriage. He looked at all of us and blushed. He sat down and started reading his paper, looking rather nervous. We looked at each other and four of us went to the toilet. We discussed the lad, saying how frightened he looked because of having to sit with us girls, and we decided to give him something to be frightened about. We would jump on him and pull his trousers off him to see him panic and squirm, then give him his trousers back. We went back to the carriage and sat down, watching him. He looked up and gave a nervous cough.

Then one of us shouted, "Get him, girls!"

We jumped on him and pulled him on to the floor. With that, the other girls joined in the fun. He never stood a chance, although he put up a good fight. Off came his trousers. He was begging us to give them back, pleading and nearly crying. A couple of girls held them out of an open window of the train, threatening to drop them.

My friend and I, who had planned this in the first place, felt sorry for him and I said, "OK, give him them back. We have had our fun!"

He looked at us a bit relieved.

They looked at us as if to say, "Who are you to tell us what to do?" Then they dropped them out of the window.

We told them off. We said, "You went too far – there was no need to throw them away. You are well out of order!"

They said, "Well, you lot started it!"

We were nearing our stop and we all got off, but the man stayed in the carriage.

While we were walking home, I said to my friend, "I wonder how he will explain to his family how he has come home without his trousers. What if the poor devil is married?"

At work we packed fancy biscuits in square tins. The drivers would fill their lorries with their orders, then ask us to throw in a couple of tins for them – which we did – and they would throw us a couple of packets of cigarettes.

Our wages were thirty shillings a week. We gave fifteen shillings to our mothers for lodgings, five shillings to our ticket man so we could buy our clothes, and we had ten shillings to spend on going out and make-up, etc.

We had been there nearly a year when our boss sent us upstairs making boxes because he trusted us to work by ourselves. He knew we would get the job done. There were three of us. We would tape up a box then send it down from our floor on a roller belt. Of course being left on our own was putting the cat among the pigeons – especially trusting me and my friend. Trouble was our middle name.

One day we grabbed the girl that worked with us. It was break time and we had to go down on to the floor below for it, we said we would send her down on the rollers and catch her below. So we grabbed her, put her in one of the boxes, taped it up so she could not get out, then sent it down the rollers to the floor below. We intended to meet her on that floor and take her back out of the box and all go through break together, but it did not work out that way. As we reached the bottom of the roller the foreman was already taking her out of the box. He had heard her yelling! My partner in crime and I got the sack. The boss asked us if we did not see how dangerous a game that was – we could have killed her. He said he had trusted us to do right by him, and we said how sorry we were, but he still gave us the sack.

We soon got another job together. We started work for Cherry

Valley Farms. They had turkeys, ducks and chickens. They did not have a canteen; they had not been in business for long, so we used to sit on haystacks with our packed lunch. We would stand by a long line that went right through the factory. The turkeys would go on a hook at the very beginning of the line, which would take the bird round the factory, where different people would do different things to the bird as it travelled through the factory.

First there were the killers. They would hang the bird on a hook and cut its throat. Then it would be dipped in hot wax and a person would pull its feathers off. Then its insides were cleaned out. Then, when it reached the other end, it would be bagged ready for the freezer. The turkeys would be running round our legs, trying to get away from the killers.

We would be picked up by the firm's bus, and on the way to work we would sing songs. One song we always sang was for the driver. He liked us singing it to him – it made his day.

SEVEN LITTLE GIRLS SITTING IN THE BACK SEAT

Keep your mind on your driving,
Keep your hands on your wheel,
Keep your dirty eyes on the road ahead.
We're having fun sitting in the back seat
Hugging and a-kissing with Fred.

One night on the way home a car was behind us full of workmen. We were in the back seat, watching and waving to them. A couple of them did a moonie at us near the car window. (A moonie was pulling your pants down and showing your bottom.) We were in stitches, pointing and laughing. Then the girls joined in the fun – they lifted up their jumpers and showed their breasts to the men. It was not long before we joined in, and half of the girls in the bus were doing it. The boys nearly crashed their car – they had to pull up quick to avoid hitting our bus. A car behind them had to screech to a stop.

The next day at work all the girls who had sat in the back seat of the bus, including me and my friend, were taken into the office. The boss told us off for showing our breasts through the bus window. We told him it was a prank everyone was doing at that time. He told us that everyone was not causing crashes, though! He sacked all of us girls who were on the back seat. Getting sacked seemed to be becoming a habit with me and my friend.

Our next job was land work. We loved working on the land – we were so fit and agile (sweet sixteen). We were picking potatoes. We each had a stint marked out for us. We would pick our marked stint, then had to wait until the tractor came round again so we could pick again.

My friend and I were so fast at it. We would help to pick a couple of baskets for whoever had their stint next to ours, and we still had time to do a couple of cartwheels up and down our stint, waiting for the tractor to come back round again.

We had done this for a few weeks when we noticed our stint getting longer and longer each day. We must have been picking four stints – our crafty ganger had been marking our stint so that it was twice as long as anyone else's. We told him to mark our stint the same as the others as we did not mind picking a couple of extra baskets, but we did mind picking a quarter of the field. He refused to mark the stints again, so we waited until the farmer came on to the field and told him we would not be coming with the ganger again and told him why.

The farmer checked the stints and told the ganger off. He told him he had no right making us pick that much just because we were quick workers. He said we should not be carrying anyone who could not keep up with the other pickers. If any potato pickers could not do their work, the ganger should not be hiring them.

He then asked me and my friend if we would like to work for him all year round instead of just seasonally. We jumped at the idea, so we worked for him full-time. He would send a Land Rover to pick us up every morning and take us home every night. We worked in most of his fields doing different land work. We would be working in one field and it would be bright sunshine, while across the road in one of his other fields it would be pouring down with rain.

The farmer gave us a hoe each to weed one of his fields. We had to tie our kerchiefs over our noses and mouths while walking up and down weeding, as the field had been spread with manure – muck, they called it. It was spread with bits of dead animals and it smelt rotten, but we got it done. We must have looked like a couple of bank robbers with our kerchiefs on. The farmer came and checked and was very pleased with us. We said to ourselves he just came to see if we could do these mucky farm jobs – he was testing us.

There was a gang picking potatoes in the next field. We had been watching them all week. When we picked potatoes the farmer would let each picker take home a small boiling of potatoes in their lunch bags. Every night when they were leaving for home we saw the ganger toss a sackful into the back of the Land Rover – he wasn't happy to just take a boiling!

As they were leaving the field one night, the farmer stopped them and made his foreman and his driver empty the Land Rover out. He pulled out the sack and emptied it on the ground, then the farmer made all the pickers empty their lunch bags of potatoes on the ground. When they had finished there were about sixteen stone of potatoes lying there. The farmer got stuck into the ganger – he told him he had really rubbed his kindness back in his face. He had allowed them to take a small boiling, and they had taken a quarter of his field. He called the ganger a thief and said he would never let him work for him ever again and would make sure no other farmer for miles around would ever hire him.

We bought ourselves a pair of boots each. I bought gold ones, and my friend bought silver. Mine had platform soles, which I had to wear, being only five feet tall whereas my friend was a lot taller. I always looked up her nose and she always told me my arse was too near the ground. Now, with my platforms, I was more or less her size. I loved it. We were meeting Teddy boys at the dance, so we decided to set our own trend: we would be Teddy girls. Some of our workmates joined us when we told them we were going to be Teddy girls – there were six of us all going to set the trend. We all went out together and bought the same gear. We bought a bird's-eye coat, which was a three-quarter-length garment with a velvet collar and velvet cuffs, three-quarter-length jeans with turn-ups, silk blouses in different bright colours, big round coloured earrings, bobby socks and suede shoes.

We all dressed like that for quite a while, and half the girls that we used to meet in the pier dance hall bought bird's-eye coats and called themselves Teddy girls.

My friend and I got fed up with being Teddy girls and went back to wearing our rock 'n' roll gear.

We decided to dye our hair one night while at my friend's house. She had black hair, so I wanted mine black; and she wanted my colour – blonde. We went and bought our dyes and did it together, following the instructions religiously. When we had finished we wrapped towels round our heads and waited for thirty minutes for the dye to work. Then we took the towels off. I nearly had a heart attack. My blonde hair had turned bright green and her black hair was now bright bottle-ink blue. My friend started killing herself laughing and I could not help laughing and pointing at her. Then we started to panic. We tried to wash it back out again, washing and rinsing a dozen times or more, but it did not budge one inch. We could not wash it back out again – it was there to stay. We were so worried. When my friend's mother came home and saw what we had done, she was hysterical with laughter. We were both downhearted – we didn't know what to do. We were so distressed, knowing we had to go to work like that – we looked like we had been dipped in ink. Mother suggested we go to work in turbans and keep our hair covered until the hairdresser could wash it out for us – so that's what we did, but we knew our workmates were going to make us suffer.

We arrived at work with the turbans on and our workmates would not leave us alone. They kept asking us what we were hiding from them under our turbans. We usually worked by ourselves in the farmer's field, but it was just our luck that this week for a full week we had to work inside the barn wriggling potatoes with about ten other land girls. We tried to tell them it was a new trend, but they were not having any of it. They said they didn't believe us one bit. They kept telling us we looked like a pair of old grannies and to take them off.

At dinner time it got the better of them. They jumped us and pulled the turbans off our heads. They were in stitches, nearly wetting themselves. That was it – we suffered for the rest of the day something terrible. They never left us alone. They made up songs and sang them: 'This Is the Story of the Green-Haired Blonde Trying to Dye Her Hair, but It All Went Wrong' and 'Ten Green Bottles Hanging on her Hair'.

They made us suffer for a full week. It was intolerable. We wanted to stay at home – we did not want to face them. We had had enough, and every time we walked into work it was "Good morning, trendies." I cannot say how happy and delighted we both felt when the hairdresser finally turned our hair back to normal. We both said to each other we would never ever dye our hair again.

Two boys we were working with asked us if we wanted to go swimming with them. We said yes and arranged to meet them at the bathing pool in Cleethorpes. We went shopping for strapless bathing costumes – we thought they would make us look more grown-up and like models. We met the boys there and they paid for us to go in. We put on our fancy costumes and sat on the side of the pool talking to them.

They asked us if we could swim, and we did not want to show ourselves up so we said, "Of course we can swim."

Then they said, "Come on, then, let's go in."

With that they ran and dived into the pool and started swimming. Me and my friend walked to the three-foot end of the pool and got in. We walked along it up to our waists and pretended we were swimming, but we had one foot on the bottom of the pool. We were hopping along, moving our arms around on top of the water. The lads came swimming up to us, diving under the water right near us. We all got out and sat talking.

They said to us, "We know you both cannot swim – we saw your feet on the floor of the pool, hopping along!"

We both blushed, bright red.

They said, "Don't worry, we will show you how to swim. It's easy – come on."

So we all went back into the three-foot end and they showed us what to do. In my case it took a while, but I managed to take my foot off the bottom of the pool.

I told my friend, "Look, I can do it – I can swim!"

She would not believe me, so I swam to the deep end with the boys. But no matter how hard my friend tried she just could not do it.

Then the lad that taught me to swim said, "I will teach you how to dive and swim underwater."

Clever clogs me agreed. He was stood in the water and I was at the edge the pool. He told me how to put my hands together and dive in and said not to worry, he would catch me. This I did, but I didn't keep my legs straight. As I dived my legs went right over my head and as I hit the water I did a bellyflop, which really hurt. I went under. When I came up I was struggling and gasping. He caught me OK, but when I looked down the top of my bathing costume had fallen down to my waist. I was showing off my bust. Everybody seemed to be looking and some whistled – especially the two boys. They were both gawping at me, their eyes swivelling. I pulled my top up and could not get out of the pool fast enough. I was so embarrassed, my face was burning hot – not that I had anything to hide. My friend followed me. We made our excuses and left the two boys there.

The next day at work the boys were telling our workmates they had seen my bust, and we had to explain to them what had happened. That was the end of our friendship with them, because they had made fun of us all day. We told our workmates they were only making fun of us because we had dumped them at the pool and they did not like being dumped, so they were getting their own back.

At least I could swim now. I tried loads of times after that to teach my friend to swim, but she never did learn how to do it.

We were working in the field, seeding, when it started teeming down with rain and blowing a right storm. The farmer took us indoors and said we could scrub the pantry shelves for him. He gave us buckets of hot water, scrubbing brushes and a mop each, then took us into the pantry and showed us some shelves to wash. He left us to it, saying he would be back later. It was a massive place, a huge basement, and one side wall was full of bottles of wine, whisky and beer. They were thick with dust. We spent a while polishing it off, but every bottle was shining when we had finished. We then scrubbed down the shelves he had shown us. When we saw another room with a door we went inside. It was a cold room, and it was full of pheasants and rabbits, all strung up on hooks hanging from the shelves. We took some of the hooks off to get to the shelves and they had maggots on them. When we got over the shock, we decided to throw them away for him because they were rotten. We put them in bags and threw them in a pit outside in the yard, which the farmer was using to burn his dirt.

We said, "That was a good thing, spotting those rotten birds. No wonder he wanted his pantry cleaning out."

We then scrubbed the cold-store shelves and mopped the floor. We were proud of what we had done because it was nice and clean.

We congratulated each other on doing a good job and thought, 'The farmer will be very pleased with us when he sees what we have done.'

When he came in and saw the polished bottles and clean shelves he said, "Nice work, girls."

We both grinned like Cheshire cats.

Then I said, "Wait till you see what we have done in the

cold room. Your birds were rotten and full of maggots, so we have thrown them in your dirt pit."

He flew into the cold room, and his face changed from smiling at us to flaming mad. He half choked on his words as he said to us, "Oh no! You have thrown away a full season's game and there won't be another shoot till next season. There was nothing wrong with them – that's how I wanted them! I would have thought you two would have known better than that. I expected you to have more sense!" His face was so angry and he said to us with a shaking finger, "The pair of you need not bother coming to work for me in the future."

We said how sorry we were and that we did not know; we thought we were doing him a favour, but he told us to go and not to bother coming back. So we did just that. Another job we loved – another sacking!

The next week we got a job in Cleethorpes in a sideshow on the beach. The beach and Wonderland was full of sideshows. Our sideshow was called 'Gloria in the Goldfish Bowl: The Little Mermaid Only Two and a Half Inches High'. My friend was sat in a box in the front taking the admission fee. I was the mermaid, Gloria (the star of the show). I was in a secret room at the back. It was a big tank full of goldfish fixed on a shelf on the wall. In the middle of the tank was a magnifying glass. I would sit on a table in front of the tank, but from the other side it looked as though I was in the goldfish tank, and tiny. I would have a bikini on and would sit on the table combing my long blonde hair, and sometimes I'd wave to whoever was watching. If I did not turn up for any reason, my boss would put his twelve-year-old son in with a long wig on.

Cleethorpes would be full of trippers, coming from Doncaster, Sheffield, Liverpool and the surrounding areas. You would be lucky if you found a place to sit on the beach in the summer.

A load of boys came in one day to see the show. They shouted out, "Hey, Gloria, we will be waiting outside for you and your friend at the front when you close. See you later, Gloria."

When we closed, which was at three o'clock, they were there. They said, "We told you we would wait for you. Come on, we will go on the cages and ghost train."

There were four of them dressed as Teddy boys, with tweed coats on with silver and gold threaded through, velvet collars, drainpipe trousers, silk shirts, suede shoes and bootlace ties with medallions threaded through. We thought they looked grand. They took us on the cages and the lads worked them up so that they went right over the top. We lasses would scream with delight. We went on the slot machines, the guns and the ghost train. Then we had fish and chips and we walked up to the castle to look out over the Humber. Then we walked them to the station because their train was due. They told us they were miners from Rossington, near Doncaster. We swapped addresses to write to each other.

A couple of months later two of them invited me and my friend to their house. They showed us the mine they worked in, took us to the pictures and around Doncaster, then took us to the station. When it was time for our train to go, the boy I had stayed with asked me if I would be his girlfriend, but I said no. I said I would still be his penfriend, but not his girlfriend. I did not really fancy him as a boyfriend, because as he was a miner he had a face full of pockmarks with bits of black coal. He wrote to me as a penfriend for about four months. In one letter he told me he was going to do his national service, and I got no more letters after that.

We were at the pier dancing one night. It was full of Teddy boys and fishermen. We loved the way the Teddy boys dressed, but the young fisher lads dressed nicely too. They would have a light-blue suit with pleats on the back, pure-silk patterned shirts and black crêpe-soled shoes. My friend and I were having a great time, rocking and rolling with the fishermen and the Teddy boys – we did not mind which, as long as they could dance. Then the fisher lads fell out with the Teddy boys because the girls were paying them too much attention and both sides decided to fight it out. Nobody could reason with them. The Teddy boys stood on one side of the dance floor and the fishermen on the other side; all the women and others not involved left the dance hall and stood outside because we knew they were going to fight it out no matter what anyone said. All the shutters went down over the bars and glasses were taken away, then they started fighting. It was not long before ambulances and Black Marias came to take them away. That was the end of our night out as they shut the pier down, just when we were having the time of our lives.

It was still early so we decided to walk along the prom to catch our bus home. All along one side of the prom were B & Bs and pubs. We were walking by one B & B, and the people staying there were sat at tables having their evening meal so we could see them through the large front windows. So we tapped on the window and they all looked at us, then me and my friend pulled our tops up and flashed our boobs at them. One bloke nearly choked on his food when he saw us, and the woman sat with him was telling him off. Her face was full of rage. He was trying not to look; he could not help himself, but he could not draw his face away. Then the next thing was that the woman smacked him across his face. He held his cheek and now his face was full of rage, but he was still looking at us. The woman jumped up out of her seat and threw the remains of her dinner at him. We ran away laughing.

We went to the Globe Picture House down Victoria Street one night because my older sister had a bet with us that we would be too scared to go. She had been the night before and said it was so frightening it had scared the pants off her. We told her that she was a big scaredy-baby and that nothing would frighten us two, so we went. It was only in the next street to ours so we were not scared. We were feeling confident. The picture was called *The Hand*, and that's what it was about – a man's hand. It would walk along the ground with its fingers. It walked up a man's body, and its fingers went round his throat, trying to strangle him, but he managed to pull it off and throw it on to a fire. He thought it would burn, but it didn't – it came back out of the fire, climbed up him again and strangled him this time. We were both terrified, but tried not to show it, acting brave to each other.

When we got outside to go home it was dark, so we were even more scared. We both ran home in the middle of the road as fast as our legs would carry us and shot into our houses. We dared not go on the pathway as there were too many dark passageways. We were thinking the hand would come out of one and get us.

When I got in my house my sister was waiting for me. She said to me, "Well, what was it like, then? Did it scare you?"

I said, "No, don't be silly – I told you I would not be frightened one bit. It did not worry me at all."

She said, "Well, that's a bit funny because you look as if you have seen a ghost, your face is so white!"

I just grinned at her, still pretending it did not bother me, and went to bed and hid my head under the covers. I never slept a wink. I was thinking the hand was crawling up our stairs. My friend told me the next day she had not slept either.

We were meeting two boys at the Winter Gardens Dance in Cleethorpes on a date, so we both went shopping for new clothes. We bought stockings each with motifs on the sides. Mine had a sailor climbing up a ladder; my friend bought a pair with birds flying up the legs. We each bought a pair of shiny red stiletto-heeled shoes and new red suspender belts.

On the day we were going to the dance to meet our dates, I started to get ready. I looked round the bedroom for my new gear, but I could not find it. I asked my older sister if she knew where my new gear was.

She said, "Yes, Avril's got them on. She is outside." (Avril is my sister who is only eight months younger than me.)

I went outside and there she was, prancing up and down the street in my nylon stockings, my suspender belt and my new shoes, showing off, swaying her hips as she walked.

I ran up to her and said, "Get them off this minute or I shall take them off you myself right here!"

She said, "No, I won't. Mother said I can wear them, so there, I won't take them off."

I said, "Mother has no right to let you wear my clothes or touch my stuff. They are mine, not hers. I bought them with my own money that I worked for. If you don't go inside and take them off I shall do it myself right here!"

She was still stubborn and said, "No, I am not taking them off for you or anyone else."

So I knocked her to the ground, undid the suspender belt, pulled off my shoes then pulled the suspender belt with my stockings and they came off all in one go, right there in the street with all the neighbours watching and laughing at us. I was right flaming mad. I marched back into the house with my gear with my sister following me, crying to Mother, telling her what I had done. I told her if she ever touched my clothes again I would give her a damn good leathering. I also told my mother never to give her permission to take my stuff again as it was me who worked hard to buy them.

She had the cheek to say to me, "Oh, you are always moaning!"

I said, "Oh, yes! How come you never allow her to touch any of the others' clothes? It's only mine, isn't it? But never mind that, just tell me what I have always thought: that I am the black sheep of this family and always have been."

I told my friend all about it and she said, "Do what I do: buy a lock and key. That will stop them touching your stuff."

So later on I did. That stopped her.

We met the boys, our dates, outside the dance, and they paid for us to go in. We danced with them for half the night and they supplied us with drinks. My friend and I were not used to drinking and we got very tipsy and felt sick, so both went to the toilet and were retching our stomachs up. We must have been in there an hour with our knees on the floor and our heads in the toilet being sick. We got our coats and caught a taxi home as we could hardly stand up, but we both got home.

The next day we both had hangovers. We were sick all day at work and we both said to each other, "Never again!" The next time we went out we stuck to Coca-Cola – we had learnt our lesson.

Our next job was in a fish factory on the Grimsby docks. We would stand alongside a moving belt, and we each had a weighing machine on a table in front of us and a kit of fish. We would cut the fish and weigh it, then put it on the moving belt for others to pack in boxes. It was so cold in there because it was full of freezers. We had to stand in buckets of hot water to stop our feet from freezing. We always had hot aches in our hands and feet and red noses. We would soak every night in our baths to wash the smell of fish away. We got used to the smell when we were together. When we went out other people could still smell it, so we changed jobs again.

Since we left school, in just over one year we had had seven different jobs. Now we started work at the ropery, making nets and rope for the trawlers. We were great friends with the boss. Because we were so fast at braiding nets, we made them for him at home then took them to work for him the next day. He would always sit with us at dinner time to give us our orders of nets to braid for him at home. Small orders or big orders, we got them done for him and we always got paid extra in our wage packets.

One dinner time he asked us if we could dance, and if we liked dancing. Of course we told him we were excellent dancers – we were bragging again as usual, but we were pretty good at rock 'n' roll in any case. He said he had a very good friend, an American, and his friend was organising a big rock 'n' roll dance for some of the servicemen and would we like two tickets? Of course we would! We nearly snatched his hand off. We loved rocking and rolling – we were always practising it every chance we had. The dance was at the Gaiety Ballroom. We would be picked up at our doors, and when the dance was finished we would be taken home again. We were so pleased.

We bought ourselves new rock 'n' roll skirts – we both had one but we wanted a new one. We even sewed lots of small bells on our frilly underskirts.

On the night of the dance we had our glad rags on and the taxi picked us up. The taxi man told us he would be outside at the end of the dance and to make sure we were there so he could take us home or he would have to answer for it. We promised him that we would, and we went inside. A doorman took our tickets and showed us to our seats. We were sat in the middle of a long table (there were two long tables on each side of the dance floor). The hall was full of American servicemen, all in uniform. Most of them did not look much older than us two – we were sixteen, and they looked a couple of years older than that. There were quite a few other girls also at our table and across the room at the other table. The servicemen's leader was sat at the end of the table. He introduced himself to us and introduced us to the lads sat at our table.

He said to them, "These two young ladies are to be your dance partners for tonight. I want you all to be gentlemen to them. They are employees of a very good friend of mine, so look after them well for me. All enjoy yourselves and have a good time."

Then he went and sat back down at the end of the table. We watched him and could see he was keeping an eye on us all night. The lads were supplying us with drinks all night – the table was full of them. My friend and I were sticking to Coca-Cola, but we did have the odd drink of beer.

Then the music started playing rock 'n' roll. Two of the men jumped up and took us by the hand on to the dance floor. They were great rockers. They were leading us and showing us how to do it their way – not that we needed any showing how to do it, but we did it like they wanted us to. We fell straight into it. They tossed us up and over their heads, and spun us round and through their legs. When the others saw how good we were, they took it in turns to dance with us. No sooner had we sat down and had a couple of sips of our Coca-Cola than we were pulled up again. Some of the young men on the other table facing us tried to muscle in, but the lads on our table had it all worked out – they never got a chance of a dance. We must have danced with all the young men at our table.

When the dance ended the lads took it in turns to thank us for their dance, picking our hand up and kissing it. Then the leader came up to us and took us to our taxi, thanking us and telling the taxi driver, "Make sure these pretty young girls reach home safely."

The taxi took us to our doors and we both said we felt like princesses.

At work the next day we were still on cloud nine.

At dinner time the boss sat with us and said, "I heard you two were the belles of the ball. My friend could not praise the pair of you enough. Said you were stars to the lads and they were honoured to have met and danced with you."

We thanked him for the tickets and told him that we had VIP treatment. Of course all our workmates were jealous of us and we could not wait to tell them where we had been.

They kept saying to us, "Yeah, you two are always creeping around the boss's arse."

We would tell them, "It's because we are his best workers."

We kept rubbing it in about what a fantastic time we had. They kept saying that is not why you are his favourites; it is because you make extra nets for him. We just started singing songs every time they started on us. We sang 'Rock Around the Clock' and 'Sweet Sixteen'. It riled them up.

My friend fancied a lad that worked on the waltzers at Wonderland, so we would go on them every time we went to Cleethorpes. They always let us on for free. Once the waltzer gathered speed he would pick one or the other of us up and hold us over his head with his arms outstretched. I was picked up most of the time – I think it was because I was small and only weighed seven stone. My friend was tall and weighed nearly ten stone, so she got away with it. He fancied her as well, but they never did go out on a date.

One day at dinner time in the canteen the girls on the table behind us were hysterical with laughter. We turned round to see why. We saw a new girl that had just started there, and we recognised her as she had been in our class at school. She saw us and came over and sat with us. Worst luck for us, as we had had enough of her when we were at school! She got us the cane many times because of what she used to do. She could fart to order, whenever she wanted to. We would say to her, "I bet you sixpence that you cannot fart five times." But she always did. The trouble was she would do it when we did not want her to. Her favourite time was when we were having singing lessons and singing our favourite song. The song was about a train trying to reach the top of a very high hill, struggling to get there. It went like this:

It was chugging along and thinking and saying,
"I think I can, I think I can, I think I can . . . "

And at that very part of the song she would sing, "To where I stood and farted." Then she would fart. We would have a job trying to carry on singing, because we could not stop ourselves from laughing. She carried on singing away, as brazen as anything, with a straight face:

"I said I could, I said I could, I said I could, I said I could,
I said, I said, I said, I said I could . . . "

We would all be laughing and sniggering, and our singing teacher would cane us for it, but he would praise her for singing on her own. We never told him it was her fault we could not sing – we were too embarrassed to tell him she had farted, so we accepted our punishment. And now here she was, still up to her old tricks, taking bets on farts. We did our best to keep away from her, but every time she managed to latch on to us we couldn't get rid of her.

Boyfriends

One day after work we went shopping down Freeman Street.

Coming out of a dress shop we bumped into a gang of young fishermen. They had just come out of the pub. We couldn't believe it – it was Robert with some fishermen friends. We hadn't seen them for eleven years. The last time we had seen him I was five and a half years old, during the war, but I still recognised him and he recognised me. It must have been fate that brought us back together again.

He told us they were deep-sea trawling and had landed that morning and were going to meet up with other fishermen off their ship in the Humber Pub to talk about their landings. He asked us to join him for a drink – so we did.

We were talking about when we last met as children, and Robert told me he often thought about me, and would I go out with him and be his girlfriend?

I agreed and told him I had wondered if I would ever see him again, and was I not supposed to be his girlfriend anyway? I had often wondered if we would ever find each other again, and now we had. My friend hit it off with one of Robert's friends and agreed to be his girlfriend.

They were both sailing on the same trawler and only had two days on shore before trawling again for three weeks. They took us to the pictures after settling up down at the dock and we promised to see them when they landed again.

We courted them until we were both seventeen, seeing them every time they landed from sea. They would tell us how their trawler would ice up so much that they would have to chop the ice off the trawler to stop it sinking, and among the things they trawled up in their nets were dead animals, a piece of submarine and bombs. They once watched a trawler turn over with the ice on it and watched the fishermen running up the side of it and the mast trying not to sink with it. They did not last long in those waters.

Robert and his friend got called up for their national service when they came home, and after their six weeks training, before being posted, we all got married.

Married

My friend's husband and Robert got posted to different camps, and she left Grimsby to live with her husband's mother in Newcastle. I never saw her again, but I heard they had one baby, a boy. So that was the end of fifteen years of friendship, but now I had Robert. I was seventeen and he was nineteen.

My mother once again told me it would not last. She was not keen on him at all because he was a Roman Catholic. Robert's mother was the same – she did not want him to marry me, she wanted him to marry the daughter of her best friend, but he told me he had never been out with her, and had never even wanted to and it would never have been. He told his mother that I was the only one for him, so she might as well accept it, and I told my mother the same. So we did not get any help from either of them. We had to make it on our own. Times were hard, but I was used to going it alone as I had always been the black sheep of the family. My brothers and sisters got any help they needed, while I got next to nothing. At least it made me hard. I always told myself I did not need anyone's help, especially now I had Robert, my husband, my soulmate, my friend. What more could I want?

Robert would sing to me every night before we went to sleep. He was so happy. A couple of songs he always sang were 'Look Homeward, Angel' and 'My Special Angel'.

National Service

We stuck together through the good and the bad. We were on our own. We did not care – we were together. He could not do enough for me.

All we ever got from our mothers was "You've made your bed, now lie in it." They were hoping we would part, but they were to be very mistaken.

Robert finished his army service and we had our first baby, a boy, but then he had to go back and do an extra eight months for all the time he had been AWOL. The reason he was always going AWOL was because he hated the army. He never wanted to go back to camp when he came home on leave, especially after our first son was born. He always went AWOL. The MP would come to take him back to camp, and Robert would talk him into letting him go back under his own steam. They would trust him, but he always let them down. They would see him off on the train at Grimsby Town Station and he would get off at the first stop, so then a couple of MPs would take him back to his camp in handcuffs.

One time when he was on leave, out shooting game with one of his cousins, he shot the end of his little finger off. I met him at the hospital.

He was grinning and said to me, "Now they won't take me back until my finger gets better."

He soon found out that would not work – the MP came and took him back, and he ended up doing his extra eight months in Colchester.

Eventually his national service ended and he went back to sea – Iceland, the Faroes, Greenland, the coast of Russia – all deep-sea fishing. He was even in the cod war – throwing their catch at the gunboats, who always cut their nets when they caught them.

We had to stay with his mother temporarily while we were waiting for a council house. My mother had no room for us as my oldest sister and my three brothers had all got married within a few months of each other, so I had to put up with Robert's mother. She had had a son late in life – he was born three weeks before our son, so he was my son's uncle. She warned me I had to say they were cousins whenever anyone asked because she did not want to say her baby was her son's baby's uncle. Our sons were ten months old and just crawling around, not able to walk yet.

When Robert came home from sea, he would always bring a bond home after each trip and his mother would always keep it. I did not say anything – we had to live with her for a while and I was already in her bad books for marrying him. After one trip he brought back a couple of big bars of chocolate.

She grabbed them off him and said, "I will sort these out later." Then she put them away.

When Robert went back to sea she took one of the bars of chocolate out, gave her son some, ate some herself, then put it away again while looking at me, sneering. I said nothing because I knew she was only looking for an excuse to throw me out on the streets the first chance she got. I did not care about her having his bond, but I thought it was evil of her to eat the chocolate in front of our baby when it was his dad's bond and meant for all of us.

She had named her son Stephen, after her friend and because she liked the name. She would leave me to mind him while she worked at the butcher's. I did not mind because the two boys loved playing together.

After Robert's second trip I was four and a half months pregnant with our second child. Robert told his mother because we were both very happy about it, but she went crackers at him in front of me, saying to him, "Oh well, you have got yourself well and truly tied up now – nobody will want you with two kids."

He went mad at her. He said, "I've told you, Mother, I have my wife. I don't want or need anyone else. I am happy with my family – I love and need them. And don't worry, we will be out of here in a few weeks so you won't have to put up with us much longer, and I for one cannot wait. I'm hoping after this trip we will be gone from here."

She wasn't very pleased with him saying that to her at all.

After he had gone away to sea, one day she said to me, "I think we will go out for a walk, just to the post office. It's only round the corner and it will give the boys some sunshine and fresh air and us two some exercise."

It was not far and I thought I might as well try to please her, so we went. Neither of us had a pushchair or pram, so we had to carry our sons as they could not walk yet. Being ten months old, my son was heavy; and being nearly five months pregnant, I was tired. When we reached the post office and were standing near to the door she pushed Stephen into my other hand so I had a baby in each arm.

She said, "Hold him – I won't be a minute. I'll be straight back – I only have to post a letter."

She rushed inside, leaving me stood there with a baby on each hip. After a while she still had not returned, so I sat on the ground so I could sit them both down. I waited and I waited and I did not feel too good as I kept getting small pains in my stomach; so I got to my feet and carried the boys home, one on each of my hips.

When I reached home I was in bad pain. I put the boys in the playpen and lay on the couch. I knew I was going to lose my baby and I had called the doctor, who was coming round to see me. Before he came Robert's mother came in. I asked her what she thought she was playing at leaving me to carry both boys home when I was pregnant. I even accused her of doing it on purpose.

She said, "Don't be silly, of course I didn't."

So I said, "Then why did you leave me holding the two heavy boys? Why did you not come straight back?"

She said, "I was going to come straight back, but I bumped into my friend, Steven, and we had a quick cup of tea. When I went back for you you had already gone."

I said to her, "Well, you will be happy to know I am losing my baby."

The doctor came in, and after seeing me he called an ambulance and I had a miscarriage.

When he came home from sea, Robert asked me what happened and I told him I had been silly to try to carry the two boys together. He went out and bought me a pushchair. He might as well have given it to his mother because she never let me use it.

That trip we got our council house. It was not very far from where his mother lived, but it was ours – a house of our own. We had another baby – a girl. We visited his mother once a week. The two boys, Stephen and my son, you could not part them. They would go travelling off whenever they got the chance, so we would have to pin their name and address on their back. The police were always bringing them back home. Stephen had a small dog called Prince. When the police van brought them home, it would stop and the back of the van would open and out would come the little dog with the two boys following. The tricks they got up to at their age (they were both only three) are unbelievable. They would wait for Stephen's father to fall asleep, then they would tie his shoelaces together; then they would wake him up by breaking an egg on his bald head, then leg it.

Robert liked a good drink and once when he had taken the two lads to Cleethorpes on the train they made him take them on all the roundabouts. He came home by taxi with them because he could not help being sick.

I was thankful that my son had a kind grandad. He was kind to all my children.

Their grandmother, well, she was a different kettle of fish to me whenever she got the chance. On one occasion we were in her house on our usual once-a-week visit. I was eight months pregnant – it was going to be a Christmas Day baby, and I only had one month to go before the birth. Robert wanted to do another trip at sea, but he was worried about who would mind our son and daughter if I went into labour before he came home.

His mother said to him, "It will be all right if she has it before you land. I will watch them for you until she comes back home after the birth."

I was worried and so was he.

She said, "Don't worry, you can rely on me. I'll have the two children until you land if I need to."

He said to her in a worried voice, "Are you sure? Because I need to know they will be safe."

She said, "Yes, you can trust me. Don't worry – they will be fine."

Robert's sister came in with her children, and after a drink and a chat together we all decided to go.

She left first and as they went his mother said to his sister's children, "Here you are – here's some pocket money each for my favourite grandchildren."

As we left she said nothing to me or mine.

When we were walking home my oldest one said, "Why didn't Nanna give us some pocket money? Isn't she our Nanna too?"

I felt so awful, I could have cried.

Robert said to our son, "Never mind. Nanna has run out of money, but yes, she is still your grandmother and I'm going to give you some money for sweets."

Robert felt it also. I hated her doing things like that to my children. She only did it to hurt me because I married her son, but it was no fault of my babies. It's a good thing their grandad loved them.

She was not that good to him either, so it wasn't just me who got her wrath. One day when we had called on her she showed us £100 that she had won at bingo.

She said to Robert, "Don't tell your father I've won at bingo as he will want some and I have bills to pay."

Robert's father came in from work. He said to her, "Can you buy me five cigarettes or lend me the money for some baccy as I haven't got a smoke. I'm gasping – I haven't had a whiff all day!"

She said to him, "Where do you think I get money from? I've got nothing."

Robert and I looked at each other in disgust. All that money and she would not buy him five cigarettes – her own husband.

Robert and I shared everything, even though we did not have much. Robert took out his packet of cigarettes and said, "Here, Dad, you can have these – I have some more at home."

His father said, "Are you sure, son?"

Robert said, "Yes, Dad, I have some tobacco and cigarettes at home."

Robert's mother sat there and did not blink an eye or say a word. Robert didn't have any more at home!

When we got outside he said to me, "I didn't know what a greedy, selfish mother I had. She has opened my eyes, that's for sure, and I shall tell her so the next time I see her. I shall let her know what I think of her."

I said, "You don't know the half of it, but it's best not to say anything as I might have to rely on her if I go into labour before you have landed. No matter what you say, it won't change her. She has always been selfish, especially to me and our children, because she does not like me. My mother was not too keen on me marrying you, but she has never done anything to ever hurt you; she has always made you welcome."

The next day Robert went to sea. He was fishing off Greenland, so he would be away longer than usual. He would never let us wave him off because fishermen said we would be waving them overboard, and I was not allowed to wear a green coat!

A week before he was to land I fell down the stairs, missing all the stairs and landing at the bottom of them. I was lying there unconscious for I don't know how long, but when I came to my son, who was three and a half years old, was stroking my face saying, "Mummy," and crying. I put him and my fourteen-month-old daughter in the pram and went to their grandmother's (Robert's mother) for help. My baby was due in one week's time, which would be Christmas Day. It was early morning and there was ice on the ground. I knew the baby I was carrying was in trouble. I got to her door and started banging on it, shouting her name. She had promised Robert she would mind the children for me. I was stood there a while – I could hear whispering.

She opened the bedroom window and said, "Yes, I know I promised to mind the children, but I have too much to do this week; you'd better go to your own family for help."

Hearing that, I walked away from there. I had to walk halfway through the town and knock for my sister, my nearest relation. Now it was snowing and blowing a gale, but she was up. She promised to mind my children for me and called me an ambulance.

The doctors tried for five hours to save my baby's life, but in the end my baby was stillborn – another girl. I was heartbroken and numb.

I had to watch all the other mothers with their babies, nursing them, and I could not stop crying. I was in there all Christmas. Doctors and nurses came round, giving us presents, but I could not be cheered up. No one could give me my baby back. The worst of it all was that I heard carol singing in the background while I was having my stillborn baby, and they were singing, "Long time ago in Bethlehem . . . " I don't think I will ever forget that carol. I never saw anything of Robert's mother – she never bothered to come and see me, which was nothing new because all the time I was married to her son she never ever came to see us; it was Robert and I that went to see her.

I was still devastated inside – who wouldn't be? I carried that baby for nine months. It was going to be a Christmas baby. Robert and I were looking forward to our Christmas baby, and now he was never going to see her. He knew her because at night she would kick him in his back – like a footballer, as he would say – so at least she made her presence known to him. I could not wait for his return home to me and our other children. He also took it badly, but life goes on.

I would play the guitar. He loved me playing it to him and there was one tune he kept asking me to teach him. He loved the tune so much he wanted to be able to play it himself. I could not read music, but I would just pick the tune out by the sound of the strings. I did not know the right words, but we always sang these, and he learnt to play it.

On wings of love I'll bear thee
Enchanting realms to see.
Come, my love, let's prepare thee
In dreamland to wander with me.
A garden I know of roses,
A silvery moonlit hour;
Upon the lake reposes
A lovely dreamland flower.
On wings of love I'll bear thee
Enchanting realms to see.

A year later we had another baby girl. She was born at home. Robert had given up the sea and worked on shore. He looked after me this time. The baby only weighed 2 lb 14 oz and she looked like a little porcelain doll. The midwife said she was tiny but healthy, so would not need to go in an incubator as she had plenty of flesh on her. When she cried it was just a little squeak.

The neighbours would always come running across to look at her, and even when she was a year old she still looked like a little doll. She had red hair, taking after me, but she had a big birthmark in the shape of a fish on her stomach – the same place and the same birthmark Robert had. My other daughter was the spitting image of her father, and my son looked like me but was to have his father's ways when he grew up.

We had another council house on the Nunsthorpe Estate now, but my son and Robert's brother remained friends for life and we still visited Robert's mother quite often.

We loved our house at Nunsthorpe. The neighbours were all free and easy, but sometimes they had street fights over nothing. After fights the youngsters would search around for what they could find, like coins, earrings and necklaces which had been lost in the fights.

Our next-door neighbours were fishermen and Robert had sailed with one of them in the past, but now my husband worked for himself. He made eel nets at home, and he and his mate would drop them in ponds and rivers to catch eels. They would box them up and send them to Billingsgate Fish Market. We had to keep the eels alive – they could not sell them if they died – so we had a shed full of baths of eels in our garden.

One night our next-door neighbour had landed from sea and everyone was in bed. The taxi dropped him off just outside his house and cleared off. He tried walking to his front door (Robert and I were watching him from our bedroom window). He kept trying to reach his front door, which was only a couple of yards away, but he was so drunk that for every step he took forward he would take a step back. We got tired of watching and went to bed. In the morning I looked out of the window. He had not made it to his front door – he was fast asleep, stuck in the middle of his hedge. His wife came out and took him inside.

He always took me and Robert and our children inside his house every time he landed from sea. He would sit the children on his fireside rug, give them a load of nuts and a nutcracker and laugh at them trying to crack them open. He would insist that Robert and I should have a drink with him and would never take no for an answer. The trouble was it was always his home-made beer – it blew your head off! I did not drink and Robert was only used to a few, but he would keep on filling our glasses up – we could not stop him. There was a long row of plants on his window sill, just behind where I was sitting, so they got my drink every time. He would brag about how well his plants were growing and how nice and green they were, so I did not feel guilty about feeding them my drink. They were thriving on it.

One of our neighbours who lived a couple of houses down was stood on the other side of my next-door neighbour's hedge. I was talking to my neighbour and she did not see us. We heard someone walking by say to her, "What are you hiding behind the hedge for? Are you waiting for someone?"

She replied, pointing to my house, "I am waiting for her daughter to come out. I am going to give her a good leathering because she has just hit my son!"

Her son was at least six years older than my daughter. She did not know I had heard and seen her.

I went up to her and said, "You're going to do what? Well, never mind about waiting to hit my daughter, just try hitting me – I'm nearer your age!"

She didn't want to know. She started running for her house. I flew after her and caught her in her backyard. I smacked her one right in her face then grabbed hold of her, throwing her to the ground. She was a fat woman, weighing about fifteen stone. I was small, weighing eight stone, but I always said, "The bigger they are, the harder they fall!" As I tried pulling her back up off the ground she fell backwards. Her round dustbin was behind her, and when she stumbled back on to it she fell with her arse stuck in the bin. She was trying to get her arse out of the bin and I was killing myself. I was in stitches, it was so funny. Then her husband came out. I was still in hysterics because of the way she was swaying from side to side with the bin still stuck on her bum. He asked what was going on.

I told him, "I smacked her one because she said she was going to leather my six-year-old child. Nobody touches my children except me and my husband!"

Even her husband was trying not to laugh. Then he said to me, "Well, if that's the case if I was you I'd finish it off and put the lid on the bin, and it serves her right!"

And he went back inside, leaving her still stuck in the bin.

If my husband had said that to me I would have gone mad. He would never have heard the last of it. The man would not have dared say anything to me anyway because he was scared of my husband – he knew that my husband would punch him.

My husband and his cousin started fishing for Dover sole as well as eels and they made enough to buy a fishing boat together, so he finally became a skipper of his own fishing boat. Up until then, when he put his nets on the beach he would take me and the children with him, and we would collect fancy shells off the beach, take them home, paint them and make all sorts of fancy things with them; now we could not go. But Robert was happy with his fishing boat. On slack days he would take anglers out to fish around the two forts in the Humber, but, after a good few years of fishing, dock fees became too dear for the pair to keep running the boat, so they sold it. My husband bought himself a small boat so he could fish on his own. That way, what he earned was his. He carried on making his own nets and still did his eels.

One day I went out with him and our son. He was showing us how to catch eels without lines – we were to catch them with wool. We sailed out onto the River Humber, dropped anchor and put our wool over the side, and it wasn't long before we were pulling up eels. My son had a weird fish on his wool, but as he tried to pull it aboard it got away. We knew what fish were in the Humber, but we had never seen a fish like that before. The eels were coming aboard quite well – they would swallow the wool and it would stick in their throats like a hook. We were all bragging to each other each time we caught one. Then I pulled into the boat the biggest eel any of us had ever caught before. It was like a conger eel.

I was so excited, I shouted out to them, "How about that then? Look at the size of it! Beat that if you can."

I had landed it in the middle of the boat and as I was looking it raised up like a snake and started dodging backwards and forwards at my legs and it sounded like it was hissing at me. It was attacking me. I panicked, and my excitement turned to fear and fright. The joy of pulling up the biggest catch of the day was gone like a flash.

I jumped on top of the cabin roof, screaming at my husband and son, "It's getting me. Get it. It's attacking me."

They looked at me and the eel and started laughing. They were doubled up with laughter, saying, "Come on down, you silly devil."

I told them, "There is no way I am coming down while that eel is still there waiting for me."

They had tears in their eyes with laughing, but I would not come off the roof, so they put it in the cabin. When I saw it safely locked away, then I got down. We then decided to call it a day and head back for the lock gates.

It was flat calm when we started out, but now it was blowing up a storm. On the way back down the river the sea was raging and going over us from all sides. Even the big trawlers were making a run for the lock gates to get safely into the docks. The small boat we were on only had a small hand engine fastened on to the back of it, and my son was trying to steer. I watched the waves going right over him and the engine – it terrified me.

We got to the lock gates and they were shut. We had to wait a while before someone would open them to let us through. We were in between the big trawlers, hoping they might give some protection from the waves, but we were still getting washed from both sides. I was praying for the gates to hurry up and open, because each time the waves came my son would disappear under them then appear again. I was sick with worry and fear.

The gates opened to let us in – the trawlers let us go in first. At last we entered the docks and my brave son, who had stayed steering the fishing boat, steered us safely into the fish docks. I was thankful we were on land. After the two of them tied up and put their eels and nets in the van we went home. I swore I would never go on a small boat ever again, and I never did go on that small boat again. I said the sea was not for me.

Robert's hobby was going game shooting with his cousin. He would fill our freezer up with pheasant, duck, geese, and fish from fishing with his small boat. He was sometimes out all night with his mate. They stayed out for the night flight and the morning flight but one day they came home with nothing. They were sat cleaning their guns when our fourteen-year-old son came in – he took after his father, always going out into the countryside with his mates and their catapults.

He said to his father, "I can see you have been out shooting, Dad. Did you get anything?"

His father said, "No, son. We stayed for two flights and got nothing."

With that the lad pulled a goose out of his bag, saying, "Well, Dad, I did! I got it with my catty."

I butted in and said, "Well, what a show-up for you two. The pair of you have been out all night for birds with your shotguns and gun dogs and come home with nothing, and your son comes home with a goose."

They said, "Trust you to show us up."

I never let them forget it. Every time they went out shooting I would ask Robert if he was taking our son out with him to show him how to get the birds. He would just laugh it off.

Robert took me to the pictures because 3-D and Technicolor had come out in our town. Everybody was queueing up to see it. It was the talk of the town. We did not think we would get in to see it because the queue was miles long (when we joined it was three streets away) but we did. We sat down to watch *Rebel Without a Cause*. Rebels on horseback were slicing off the heads of soldiers they were fighting and vice versa. As they cut a head off it would come flying out of the screen straight at us and the bright-red blood seemed to spray on us. Women were screaming and fainting. Ambulances kept coming outside, taking people with weak hearts out of the picture house, because like us they had never seen anything like this before and it shocked them. We still had black-and-white television. Robert and I thought it fantastic.

My big, brave husband, Robert, took me out shooting with him in the countryside. He was going to meet his mate there. We arrived at a field which was full of cows and a big bull.

He said, "Come on, we will take a shortcut through it."

I hesitated. I said, "I don't like the look of that big bull. It looks mad and it's got a big iron ring through its nose. I don't like the idea of going past it or the cows."

He said, "It will be all right as long as we ignore them and do not run. We won't frighten them and they will ignore us. I will walk in front to protect you in any case."

He managed to get my trust after a lot of umming and ahing, so we went through the gate, him walking in front. I closed the gate, lagging slowly behind him. We must have got about a quarter of the way into the field when the bull started coming towards us with the cows following it. I panicked with fright. I looked at Robert to say something, and I couldn't believe it – he was gone. All I could see was a cloud of dust. He was running so fast for the other side of the field, like lightning. He always was a fast runner, but that's the fastest I've ever seen him run. That was greased lightning. My mouth dropped open – I was flabbergasted. I could not say anything. The bull and cows were running after him, but he reached the other side. There was a wire fence about four feet high and it was electrified to keep the cows in the field. He tossed his gear over it with his gun and leapt over it himself, clearing it without any trouble. I ran back to the gate, went through it and made sure I shut it in case they came back for me. I walked around the edge of the field to where Robert was waiting for me. When I approached him he was grinning at me.

I said, "Well, thanks for that show of bravery. Thanks for you protecting me. You had the cheek to tell me not to run, and all I got from you was a trail of dust!"

He laughed at me.

When we met up with his mate I told him what Robert had done. Robert told him he had done it on purpose – he could see he had riled the bull, so he drew its attention from me and put himself in danger so I could get away safely. He said if we'd stayed together he knew we both would not get over the fence before the bull got to us. I didn't know whether to believe him or not as no one could argue about that.

My eldest daughter was a daddy's girl. She was the spitting image of Robert. She was the one who sat on his shoulders. It was always "Can I have a piggyback?" She never walked if he was with us. She would always take the mickey out of him because he had a big nose – we all took the mickey out of his family because they had big Roman noses.

Our daughter would always say to him every time she was on his shoulders, "You'd better keep hold of me tight, Dad, because I might slide down your nose."

He would always reply, "Are you taking the piss out of your old dad, you cheeky little monkey? If you don't be careful I will make you walk."

When she was a toddler she went and smashed one of his front teeth out. He was fast asleep on the sofa, and she was playing with her pottery doll and pram. She took the doll over to her dad to show him, but he just snored and carried on sleeping. But he soon woke up because she brought it down on his face, saying, "Dad, Dad, Dad!" That day he was less a front tooth, which was a terrible shame because he had a beautiful set of teeth and a wonderful smile. Now he had to have a false one.

After that if he was ever nasty I would say, "If you don't shut up I'll get our baby daughter to knock the other teeth out for you."

He would smile and say, "Oh, very funny!"

Or I would swear at him because he hated to hear women swear. My children knew this and never dared swear in front of him. He thought they never did swear and would always praise them up for it, but I knew different because I had heard them swearing to their friends outside. He never knew half of the tricks they got up to, especially the boy.

One day I thought I would have a nice soak in the bath, so went into the bathroom to fill the bath up. When I looked into the bath it was full of water with a big stone in the middle. I must have jumped a foot in the air with fright because a big toad jumped up out of the water and sat croaking at me, jumping on and off the rock.

I shouted out to my son, "All right, you can come up here right this minute and clear this lot out before your father gets home. He will want a bath and so do I!"

I was always getting shocks like that because my son was wildlife mad, like his father. He would bring a fox home or a duck or even hedgehogs.

He always said, "Mam, I have found them outside. They are lost and have no mother or a home to go to."

One day it was a poisonous snake.

My husband Robert said to me, "There is only one poisonous snake in Britain and our son has to find it, doesn't he?"

Another time I thought I would clean our son's bedroom dresser. I opened the drawer and out flew a jackdaw. Then I went to wash my hands in the sink and there, swimming around, was a big black lizard. In the shed, perched on a tree branch, was a barn owl. He was only small, our son, but he had put half a tree in that shed for that owl.

One day a policeman came knocking on our door and said, "Your son has been in an accident and is in the hospital. He has been knocked off his bike by a car."

The policeman then gave my husband and me his bike.

134

We took one look at it and saw it was mangled. My husband fainted and I nearly did. We thought the worst had happened. The police could not tell us what state he was in; they had just been told to let us know that he was in the hospital. We dashed to the hospital, not knowing what to expect. My husband was in a worse state than I was. He always fainted if the children ever hurt themselves.

When we walked into the hospital a doctor took us to see him. He was sat up on a stretcher, laughing and joking with one of the ambulance men, who told us he only had a badly sprained foot, which was all bandaged up. Then he told us that when he reached the scene of the accident he saw the state of the bike mangled up in the middle of the road, and our son was lying sprawled on the road near the car on his back, unconscious. The driver was very distressed, thinking he would die. His chest was going up and down and moving about. They feared the worst. When paramedics lifted his jumper up, out popped a bedraggled chicken, and when our son regained consciousness he told them he had found the chicken walking down the lane and it was lost. He did not know where the chicken lived. It was homeless.

With the things that boy got up to I don't know how my husband and I survived. When I used to ask Robert to tell him off, he would always say, "He is only a child and boys will be boys. I was the same at his age – eleven years old."

One day the police came to tell us our son had been shot in the face. That was another time we nearly had a heart attack. When we got to the hospital he was being X-rayed. They told us they were seeing where the pellets were so they could take them out.

My husband had tears in his eyes. He was trying hard to hold it together and so was I. We both felt sick with worry. The nurse told us he and his friends had been messing around with airguns. After a long wait a doctor told us the pellets were too dangerous to remove because of where they were. One was too near his brain and if they tried to remove it he could die, and another was stuck in his brow and if they tried to remove it he might go blind, so they decided they would not operate.

Days later when he came home my husband told him not to mess around with guns ever again as he did not ever want a scare like that again, but the lad never stopped shooting with his friends and later he got shot again. This time it was in his foot while out shooting vermin with his friends. As his father said to me, what could he say to him about having guns when all his life he himself would go shooting?

Robert and I often went out into the countryside or to the seaside and just sat there watching the waves crashing on to the shore. We did this one night and on the way back home Robert was smoking away while driving. He was puffing away on his cigarette and talking when he dropped it on the floor. Not thinking, he took his hands off the wheel and stooped down looking for it. I couldn't believe what he was doing.

I shouted at him, "Get hold of the wheel!"

But it was too late. We bounced off the road and ended upside down in a field. Luckily we were both unhurt and managed to get out of the car.

We tried to push the car over, trying to get it back the right way up, but we couldn't, so we left it and walked home. Robert took a couple of his mates with him to get his car back. They came back later with it, and although it was a bit battered it was still running all right. He banged a few dents out of it, saying it would last him a few years yet.

Another time I went out into the countryside for a ride with him we skidded and landed on top of a bank. The car was balanced half over the edge of the bank. I looked down and it was about a fifteen-foot drop to a river running below us. The water looked deep and it looked like a strong current. We sat there and froze. We dared not move in case the car slid down the bank into the water below us. We were both silent.

I was getting ready to panic when Robert spoke first. He said to me, "Move over very slowly to the door, your side. Open it slowly and get out on to the bank top."

I did what he said. I edged along my seat slowly, hoping the car would not move. I opened the door and got out slowly. I crawled up on to the bank top and moved away from the car. I was terrified in case Robert and the car slid down the bank. I walked around to Robert's side of the car to open the door for him. As soon as it opened he dived on to the bank top alongside me. We were both relieved. We sat there watching it, thinking it was going to go, but it did not. It stayed there, not moving. I'm sure if we had blown on it it would have gone over the edge.

I said to him, more jokingly than anything, "Well, another fine mess you've got me in and another time I have to walk home."

We both laughed, more relieved than we could say.

His mate took him back and they tied a rope to the car and pulled it back off the top of the bank, none the worse apart from a little wear and tear.

Robert was telling his mate how we had got out of the car while it was balanced, and his mate was laughing about it until Robert said to him, "Now tell my wife how I bought her a big bunch of flowers on the way home and you nicked them off me and gave them to your wife!"

Those two were always doing things like that to each other.

When his mate was leaving to go home I said, "For nicking my flowers that my husband had got for me, I hope you get a puncture in two of your tyres on your way home!"

He laughed and left. About ten minutes later he walked back in the door.

Robert said to him, "What's up, mate?"

He said, "It's your wife. Do you know that she is really an old witch! I only got round the corner and what happened? I got a puncture in two of my tyres!"

Robert and I could not help laughing – we were doubled up.

He said, "It's your turn to help me now, mate. Just think, if I could trust that old witch of a wife of yours I would make her mend them. She is to blame, the old witch."

From then on he always called me the old witch.

Robert went with him to mend his tyres, and as he left I said, "Next time you come round here you'd better have a bunch of flowers with you to replace mine that you stole off my husband or I will cast further spells on you."

The next time he called on us he gave me a big bunch and said, "They are bigger and better than the ones he got you, so can we now call a truce?"

So I said, "Yes, I won't curse you any more as long as you never do it again."

He looked worried – I think he believed that I really was a witch.

One night my son caused a big fight. He was arguing with a lad across the road. My son was too much like his father: they didn't argue, they settled it with a punch. He shot across the road to do this. He jumped our wall then fell on his backside. He got straight up and ran to the lad and punched him one. The next thing he was surrounded by at least six lads and five women, who had come out to have a go at my son. The lads all surrounded him and were throwing punches at him. Robert ran over to help his son, but the women all started on him. He ended up on his back with all the women on top of him, lashing out at him.

I thought to myself, 'I bet he loves that!'

I grabbed a boat oar that was near the door and ran out with it, swinging it around at the gang of lads that were punching my son. I saw them drop to the ground one at a time as the oar hit them, knocking them unconscious, until there was only one lad left. Then I stopped swinging the oar, thinking I would let my son deal with him.

Later on my son said, "Next time you come to help me make sure you don't get me as well, because you even hit me with that oar."

I looked at my husband. He was still on the ground with the women on top of him, still having a go at him. Then the police arrived. They took the lads away in their van and sent the women home, telling them they would get carted off as well otherwise. They let me, my husband and son go with a warning to keep the peace.

A couple of days later it was in the paper. All the lads had been charged with causing an affray and all had heavy fines. One of them told the court that he was not fighting; he was just trying to get away from a mad woman who was knocking them out with a boat oar. He was told that was no excuse and he would still get the same punishment as all the others.

My husband's father died. My children and I loved him because he had been a good, kind grandad to them over the years. We went round there to see if his mother needed any help – Robert asked her if there was anything he could do to help her.

She said, "You can come to stay with me until he gets buried. But I only want family; I don't want anyone else."

He said, "OK, me and my wife will stay a couple of days."

She said, "Oh, no, I only want you, not your wife."

She still did not like me after all these years of being married to her son and bearing his children. I did not want him to miss out on his own father's funeral, so I told him to go and stay with her, which he did. I thought to myself, 'If I don't qualify as family now, I never will in her eyes.' But over the years nothing I did or said ever changed her, and when all is said and done she was his mother. I knew she did not have long with her health; and we only have one mother, so it's best to do what you can while they are still around, which she wasn't for much longer after.

My oldest daughter was making us grandparents soon – the daddy's girl. She now lived next door to us, and my youngest daughter lived four houses further down the street. My son was still living with us. So now I was to be a grandmother in my thirties, I told my daughter I was going to make them call me Nanna. I said I was going to give them an ultimatum when they were old enough to understand, which would be, if they call me Granny instead of Nanna they would be getting no presents for birthday, Christmas, etc. I did not mean this, of course, but over the years it worked. Robert was different: even though he was still young, he loved being called Grandad.

I went with my eldest daughter and was there at the birth – my first grandchild. I was so excited, but I wish I had never gone as she brought the place down.

My next-door neighbour said to me, "I heard her yelling – the whole street must have – and we are a block away."

My daughter had a beautiful girl.

I told my neighbour, "If she has another I shall be catching a train out of here so that I am as far away as possible. Once bitten, twice shy!"

But I never did, because when she gave birth to her second child, a son, I made the mistake of being there too. It was worse than the first time. I could not calm her down.

She terrified me as she was screaming to the midwife, saying, "Give me the needle. I want to die. I don't want it."

I was saying, "It is a bit late now for that."

I felt sorry for all the other mothers giving birth, having to listen to her saying things like that. Her boyfriend was there until he legged it – I found out later he had run all the way to the Nunsthorpe Tavern, still with the blue plastic covers on his shoes and blue hairnet on his head. I should have run with him if I had known what was coming. Because I felt so sorry for my daughter, I had labour pains. I had heard of such things, but I had not believed it until now. I was taken into another room to suffer alone. I knew when she had given birth because my pain stopped. When I went back into the labour room my grandson had been born.

When, a few years later, my youngest daughter had two sons, and my son had a daughter, I never made the mistake of being at any of their births.

So now Robert and I had five grandchildren, and my oldest daughter – the daddy's girl – lived next door to us. Now her daughter was grandad's girl. She always followed him around. Robert would be busily making his eel nets in our back garden, singing away so happily, and she, the daddy's girl, would be pegging her clothes out next door on her line. Then she would sneak up with her hosepipe and drown him. They were always trying to outwit each other. After she would drown him, he would wait a couple of days, until she had forgotten about it or was thinking she had got away with it, then he would fill up our bath with cold water and wait for her to call in on us, which she did every day. He would grab hold of her hair and drag her upstairs and throw her in it, or sometimes, while she was busy gardening, he would sneak up on her and she would get the bucketful of water thrown over her. They never did get the better of each other, but it was a very happy place.

I was working nights at a lumpers' canteen on the fish docks and my son was living with us at the time. My husband still had a small fishing boat and would go away fishing for two days at a time. As I worked nights I slept nearly all day.

One night, while at work, my manageress said to me, "You have a funny husband, haven't you? Is he a bit of a nutter or an idiot or something?"

I said, "You what? What the hell are you talking about? My husband is no nutter. Why don't you explain yourself?"

She said, "Well, one of the lumpers who lives near you saw your husband running out of your house in the nuddy the other night while you were here working. He also ran round the block naked."

I said, "Well, that's a stupid lie because there is no man in my house and there has not been for a week. My husband is on his boat fishing and I saw him sail off." I was so mad at her I got stuck into her. I said, "There is only one mad nutter and idiot in this town and that is you. My husband has not been home for days – he's doing his nets at sea. There is only me and my son in our house. And you want to be very careful what you say about people – you are liable to get your face smacked in." I was so mad.

She said, "Sorry, the lumper must have made a mistake about what house the man ran out of."

I said, "Well, you want to make sure you get your facts right in the future before you open your big mouth again, accusing people."

The next day I told my son what she had said to me. I told

him I nearly smacked her one for saying that about his father when he was not even home to defend himself.

My son shocked me. He said, "Mother, she is right: someone did run out of here in the nude the other night. It was my friend Robbo. We had a bet that he dare not do it, but he did."

Robbo was much older than my son. My son was fourteen; his friend was in his twenties.

I said, "Well, that's nice, isn't it? I called her a liar and a mad bitch and now I find out she was not. I dare not let her know she was right because she already makes my life hell. She is so nasty and hard to put up with at the best of times."

So I kept quiet about it.

Another time the pair of them played one of their pranks on me. I was in a deep sleep from working all night and I was suddenly woken up by someone shaking my shoulders. I opened my eyes, still half asleep, and there staring at me was the most horrific ugly face I had ever seen. I went into instant shock. I could not breathe, I was gasping for air and I had a deep pain in my chest. I thought I was having a heart attack – I thought I was dying.

Then someone was shouting at me. It was my son. He had snatched a mask off his face and was shouting out to me, "It's me, Mum, your son. It is only me. It's just a mask. It's a joke. It's me. It's all right, it's only me."

He knew he had gone too far this time. He knew I could have had a heart attack and I could see my reaction had frightened him. He swore on his life he would never do anything like that again. He said it was him and Robbo having bets again. I was a while getting over that and I did not sleep for days.

My grandchildren loved living near us and we loved them being near also, but every time the ice cream van came they ran straight into our house to me. And they knew they had to call me Nanna, because sometimes they would say, "Grandma – oh, I mean Nanna – can we have an ice cream?"

For a joke I would say, "You don't live here; you live next door. Go ask your mother."

They would always say, "Mother always tells us he only rings his bell when he has no ice cream left."

Then I would say, "And I have no money left!"

They would say, "Nanna, pull our other legs, they have bells on."

They soon learnt how to get round us – we loved the way they came straight to our house first.

I would love to watch children's films like *One Hundred and One Dalmatians*, *The Jungle Book*, *Cinderella*, etc., so when one was showing at the cinema I would ask the grandchildren if they would like me to take them to see it.

They would say to me, "Nanna, don't you mean that you want us to take you to see it?"

It would cost me sweets and an ice cream.

Sometimes my two daughters would say to their father, "We are off dancing and taking Mother with us. We will look after her. She could do with a night out."

So he would babysit while we went together.

On the way out they would say to their father, "Don't worry, we will make sure she picks a good-looking man to dance with."

He would look a bit worried and say, "You two, make sure you look after your mother for me."

They would answer, "We will try to sell her for a pint or even a half-one."

One night when we went dancing my daughters were to meet their boyfriends there, inside, as they would pub-crawl all the way to the dance and would be quite drunk before even getting there. So we got inside and bought ourselves a pint of shandy each while waiting for them to arrive. We just sat down and were about to take a sip of our drinks when their boyfriends walked up to us. They had had a good skinful, as they usually did.

My eldest daughter's boyfriend approached, saying, "Oh, there you are."

With that he picked her up, lifted her above his head then dropped her. She hit the floor with her head. An ambulance came to take her to hospital, and I climbed into the ambulance with her. I was mad because I hadn't even had one sip of my full pint of shandy. Her boyfriend kept trying to get into the ambulance with us, but the paramedics wouldn't let him, telling him he was too drunk. They managed to shut the door and drive off without him.

I thought, 'Thank goodness they left him behind! He has done enough damage already.'

We reached the hospital and when the paramedics opened the ambulance door I couldn't believe who was stood waiting for us – her boyfriend.

I said to him, "How the hell did you get here before us?"

He had got a taxi. He said he needed to be with his girlfriend as he was responsible for her accident and was concerned for her.

The doctor told me she was concussed and had to stay in hospital for twenty-four hours, so I left her boyfriend with her, thinking the nurse would soon sober him up.

He was always picking the girls up over his head. He and his mate were over six feet tall. Usually he would run with them and plonk them on top of a hedge, leaving them to get back off it. I don't know what his mother thought when he returned home after a night out with us, because he went home in such a state. One night he spent a full night dancing with the sole hanging off his shoe – he danced all night with it flapping about. He always lost the buttons off his shirts because he would catch his shirts on the hedges that he threw the girls on and he would be covered with scratches off them.

Another time on the way to the dance we were waiting for a bus when three of the girls wanted a wee and could not wait. There was an alleyway next to a shop, so they went down it to have their wee. Meanwhile a queue had gathered for the bus. I was at the front of it, still waiting for the girls who were down the alley. I looked down on the path and there were trails of water running down from the alleyway. People were stepping over them to get on the bus, which had just come. When the lasses came back out we all got on the bus, killing ourselves with laughter because I told them that I had told the shopkeeper they were having a wee down his alley. I told their father what they had done.

Going to the dance on another occasion, we had all gone inside a shop to buy fags. The step of the shop was thick with ice. I had a pair of white knee-length boots on with a bit of a heel, and as I came out the girls were waiting outside the shop for me to follow. I stepped over the doorstep and I skidded and skated along the path on one leg. My other leg flew up in front of me and I fell on my backside on the ground. I lay there on my back, winded. My two daughters were killing themselves with laughter, holding their sides, with tears in their eyes. They could not speak with laughing so much. I was sprawled out, still on my back on the ground, trying to get back up off the icy floor, and every time I tried to stand I fell again because my boots would not grip on the ice.

I said, "All right, you two, just carry on laughing. It doesn't matter if your mother might have broken her foot or her back. Don't help me up off the floor – just keep laughing!"

When they had pulled themselves together they helped me up. They said sorry, but they could not help laughing because of the way I skidded down. They would have defied anyone not to laugh in hysterics after seeing that. Half the night they had to stop themselves from laughing.

Robert bumped into a couple of friends he had sailed with, but now he had been working on land for twenty years. Everybody used to say the sea always calls a true fisherman back to it. I left him to go for a drink with them – I thought they would be talking about old sailing times. When he came home later that night he told me he had signed on and was going back to sea just for one trip and was sailing the next day. I was worried, but I could not stop him, even though I wanted to because his asthma was much worse now with his age. I had seen him crawling on his hands and knees to get outside for air before today, but he told me not to worry because the sea air was good for him – he could always breathe more easily at sea. So he sailed away.

He had been at sea for two weeks when his younger brother came round to my house. He was also a fisherman and his ship had just landed. He told me that before he landed he heard over the ship's radio that a fisherman had been taken off a trawler in a coma and was not expected to live. The skipper had told him it was his brother, Robert. He also told me Robert had been airlifted to Norwich Hospital. It was the first I knew about it because it had taken place in the middle of the night and it was now the morning after.

I arranged for a friend to take me there. When I got to see a doctor in the hospital to find out what was going on, and what condition Robert was in, he told me it had been a dramatic sea rescue. It was late at night, dark, and the helicopter and the crew had to take him off the trawler in the perilous seas. Robert was in a coma because of a bad asthma attack and it had been touch and go. The helicopter crew had risked their lives to save him, because each time they tried landing on the trawler they kept getting smashed against it, but they got him off in the end.

Robert was now awake from his coma. I was taken to him. He was attached to an oxygen pipe and full of wires, but he was able to talk to me. He told me what he could remember about what happened. He said he kept waking up now and again and kept thinking he was dead. He said he went up in a spacecraft full of lights in the dark and that an angel kept trying to wake him up in the sky. I explained it was the helicopter rescue crew that had taken him off the ship while he was in a coma.

After a couple of weeks he was back home.

He said to me, "That's my lot – I'm never ever going to sea again. That's my calling card."

His younger brother came round to see him. He told Robert how the rescue had been reported on his ship's radio just before he docked and he thought Robert was dead.

Robert said, "I nearly was. That is me finished with the sea forever."

His brother said, "Every fisherman says that, but the sea is in their blood."

But that was Robert's last trip – he never went back to sea again.

Robert said to me one day, "Teach me to rock 'n' roll and I will go dancing with you when you go with the girls."

So we put on some rock 'n' roll records and started showing him how to do it. He did it well and was pleased with himself.

Then I said, "Now I will show you how to spin me around."

We danced side by side, then it came to him spinning me around. He grabbed hold of my hand and pulled me to him with such force, but kept hold of my hand instead of letting go. I spun around all right! I went up in the air, did a somersault over his head and landed on the floor, shoulder blade first. I felt and heard it snap. He helped me up off the floor, but my arm had come completely out of its socket – it was hanging down loosely. I was in great pain.

He took me straight to the hospital, where a surgeon took a look at it. He said that he would fetch another surgeon to have a look, which he did. One surgeon stood looking at it from the front while the other one was behind. The one behind was feeling my shoulder and my arm.

He said, "Yes, the ball has to go back into the socket."

Before I realised it, the surgeon in front of me picked my arm up while the surgeon behind pushed it. There was a click and the pain was gone. In two seconds flat they had put my arm back in place. It was hanging correctly, and we went home.

I opted out of teaching Robert to dance. I told him someone else could take the punishment he dished out. I told him the only dance I would be doing with him again would be a smoochy one – he was never one for dancing anyway.

Robert liked shooting and training gun dogs. He took me out with him and one of the dogs he had trained. He was a springer spaniel. The children had spoilt him somewhat – he would sing with them. That dog was one of Robert's favourites also. He had a mind of his own. That day Robert opened the back door of the van for the springer to get in, but he refused. I was just getting into the front when the dog shot past me and jumped on to the front seat. Robert told him to get out, but he would not move – he had no intention of getting out. As far as he was concerned that was his seat. Robert picked him up and threw him in the back. The dog sulked all the way there.

When we got there Robert shot a duck. It fell down and landed on a bank that was surrounded by deep water. The springer would usually run straight to it, but he refused to go.

Robert kept telling him, "Bring it here."

After some time the dog swam across, picked the duck up and shook the duck from side to side, looking at Robert, then dropped it on the ground with a look that said, "If you want it, come and get it yourself!"

Robert kept shouting at him to bring it over, but he just kept picking it up, shaking it and dropping it.

Robert was flaming mad by now. The springer was looking at him and he looked like he had a grin on his face.

Robert said, "It's no good – he is still sulking because I took him out of the front seat. Now he won't do anything for me. It's no good telling him any more – I know when I'm beat. We will get in the car and drive off – he will come if he thinks we are leaving him."

So we drove off. We did not get very far before he swam back with the duck. We stopped and Robert got out of the van. The dog dropped the duck at his feet. Robert opened the back door for him to jump in, but he refused, he ran away up the field, rolled in a patch of cow manure then jumped in a pond full of black oil. He then tried getting in the van, but Robert was not going to let the dog spread that cow manure and oil all over the van, so he put the dog in a black bin bag with only his head sticking out, so he could breathe easily, and drove the dog home like that. We scrubbed him with Stardrops carpet cleaner and Handy Andy, and he came up a beautiful shiny bright colour. His coat was liver and white. All Robert's friends wanted to buy him, but he was really a family pet.

Robert, his mate and I went out on his small boat to drop some eel nets on a sandbank on Cleethorpes Beach. When we reached the sandbank it was already beginning to cover over, but we managed it. Robert and I jumped into the boat first because we only had wellingtons on and the tide was nearly up to the top of our boots. His mate had a duck suit on, so he would be the last to get on the boat, but soon the tide had reached over his waist and he was jumping up and down with each wave, so he shouted to Robert to throw him a rope to help him into the boat. So Robert threw him a rope. The only trouble was he threw him both ends of it!

His mate shouted, "You stupid idiot! I expected you to keep hold of one end to pull me in."

With that a wave knocked him off his feet. Robert and I started to panic as we watched his mate. The air was trapped in his duck suit, so he looked blown up like a balloon. He was on his back and the tide was taking him quickly to the shore. Robert started the engine and we followed him. The tide landed him on the beach first and we landed just behind him. We helped him to his feet. When we found out he was all right we all burst out laughing and talking about how funny it had been. But his mate said he would never ever ask Robert to throw him a rope again if he was in trouble because he was too thick to hang on to one end.

Robert had had enough of working for himself, so he got a security job on shore at the fish docks. He said he was feeling his age – he was sixty-one. He worked shifts, which was fine by me because I also worked shifts. He liked his job and would tell me about things he had done. When he was working nights he would stop his van in the same place on the docks to eat his lunch, and a fox would come up to his van and share his sandwiches. So I had to prepare two packed lunches – one for Robert and one for the fox. It didn't matter what was in the sandwiches – the fox ate them anyway.

One morning when Robert came home from work he said, "My friend the fox was not there last night. I reckon she's found another friend with better sandwiches than mine, or else she has been run over."

I could see he was upset about it.

I said, "Don't worry, she will be back, I'm sure of it."

Months later, when we had forgotten all about it, one morning he said to me, "I had a visitor last night. My friend the fox came back to see me and she brought two baby foxes to show me. She was walking around my van to show them off. They all got stuck into my sandwiches."

I said, "I told you she would be back. I knew it. She did not come to see you because she must have been having her babies."

She carried on showing them off to him. Then Robert was transferred to Immingham Dock so he didn't see them any more.

I always played the guitar – I taught myself when I was very young. I also used to play the piano accordion from the age of seven. I have never read music – I would just listen to a song and play it by ear. Robert loved listening to me play. He would always ask me to teach him a tune on it. I did in the end and it must have taken him six months, but he managed it. I was sorry I taught him, because I got that same tune played to me every time he had time to play it.

I had been trying for years to get him to come on holiday with me, and in the end he did. We took one of our grandaughters with us (my son's daughter) and her friend. They would go fishing with him every day, catching tiddlers, then they would come back to the hotel room and the two girls would help him to cool his bald head off under the air conditioning.

One morning I was up waiting for Robert to come home from work, but he never came. One of his workmates came instead. He told me they had taken Robert to hospital with chest pains. When I got to the hospital he was having X-rays. After a few more X-rays they told him he had terminal lung cancer.

I felt like I had been hit by a lorry – I was going to lose the only one who had been good to me, the love of my life, my soulmate, the father of my children and our protector.

Over the next few weeks he fought hard against it, but it took its toll. He ended up in a wheelchair and on morphine.

When he was stuck in hospital he asked the doctors if there was anything they could do for him; and they said they wished they could, but there was nothing.

So he told them in that case he might as well spend the rest of his time at home with his family around him. So we were all with him any chance we got. I carried on working even though I did not want to, but I knew that when I was left on my own I would still have to look after myself and run a house.

My eldest daughter – the daddy's girl – stayed and looked after him every day and nursed him so she could spend precious time with him. In the nights and on my days off I would take him in his wheelchair down to the River Freshney so he could spot the fish and wildlife. At nights I would sit and play my guitar for him. He loved that. His son would take him out for rides in the countryside, which he could not get enough of.

When we lost him we were all devastated. The children had lost their dad, who had loved them all their lives – the one who would have given his life for any one of them, including me. He had protected us all and did the best he could for us.

Even though we had been told there was no hope we didn't believe it. I felt like my life was gone. I knew I would never love anyone again and I would never forget him, but life goes on. We all have to live our lives, no matter what. We have to be strong for family left behind.

He had a Catholic funeral in St Mary's Catholic Church. He had gone to St Mary's Catholic School for all his schooldays. He left from his home, which is what he wanted. He was with me for two days before his funeral. I lit candles and kept going to him, holding his hand. It always felt warm. I would sing to him, because all through our life every night he would sing to me.

All the children were with him when he died. That is what he wanted.

Two of his funeral songs were 'For Those in Peril on the Sea' and 'You'll Never Walk Alone' – very fitting as he was a deep-sea fisherman for most of his life and he did brave the sea and all the perils of it to provide for me – his wife – and his children.

I carried on working. Life goes on and I had bills to pay. At least I had three wonderful children and grandchildren. I would never have a special love again – you only have one love in your life and I had already had mine. All my children were grown-up with children of their own, all married and settled down, with their own lives to lead.

I hated being alone, especially at night. I needed someone, if only for a companion. I couldn't bear the thought of being on my own for what life I had left.

I met Francis, a Scotsman. He had lost his wife to cancer also. He was so easy to get on with and a good man. So four years after Robert died I married Francis.

Francis had been in the army for twenty-three years from the age of seventeen. He was on Christmas Island and as a soldier of twenty he had to watch the atomic bomb go off. He was also in Singapore, Germany and Northern Ireland. Then he did fifteen years as a prison officer down south. He would tell me he had to escort many famous murderers to the courts. But now he was retired, so I retired.

He had a yacht, a catamaran, so we decided to sail to Scotland on it, sell our houses and settle up there.

So after we sold up we went to live on the yacht, which was moored in Dover, to get it ready for our journey to Scotland. We spent a couple of days looking around Dover then set sail for Grimsby docks – the first stage of our journey. We sailed to the Norfolk Broads. We couldn't get too far down the Broads because our mast was too high, but we spent a few days there. Then we set sail for the River Humber, our next stop. After about five hours' sailing we realised we were not getting very far – we were making no headway. The tide was pushing us back. If anything we were just moving a little forward and then being swept further back.

Francis checked his engines. On a catamaran you have two engines and two hulls. It was then he found out one engine was not working. He tried everything, but nothing worked. He could not steer the yacht. We were not going anywhere, so he tried the sails. I had my eye on an object on the shore, and every time we seemed to get level with it we were taken backwards again. Then we had to take the sails back because by now it was blowing up a storm. It got so bad we had to call out the lifeboat because the storm was throwing us around. We had no control of the catamaran at all – we were just getting tossed about.

The lifeboat came to our rescue. They threw Francis a line so we could secure our yacht to the lifeboat. They had to throw him the line a few times before he caught it and secured us, because each time they tried this the sea would cover him. One of the crew winched himself on to our yacht. He tried the engines, but no joy, so they towed us to a harbour called Wells-next-the-Sea.

We had some cans of beer on board, so Francis and the lifeboatman were drinking them and showing off to the lifeboat crew that were towing us in. Meanwhile it had got around onshore that the lifeboat was towing in a crippled yacht to Wells-next-the-Sea, and as we reached the harbour I looked through the cabin window and there stood all along the harbour wall were about forty people – a welcoming committee, all lined up waiting to see who was being towed in. As we landed and tied up, it took me all my time to come out of the cabin and face them. I felt so stupid and embarrassed, but the crew just about dragged me out, saying we had to take them all to the pub for a drink. The pub was in the harbour. As Francis and the lifeboat crew member had been tormenting them, they thought it fit that he owed them. After all, it was them that had saved us by towing us in.

As we walked by all the people that were lined up, I had my head down. I did not look up.

Then one of the crew said to me, "Hold your head up, then." And he took hold of one of my hands, held it high in the air and shouted out, "This is Madonna!"

I pulled my hand away and felt even more stupid. We went into the pub and stayed drinking with them, buying them beers and whiskies to thank them for saving us.

Francis always contributed to the lifeboats every month, so everyone was happy.

We spent a few days there while Francis was having the engines mended. It was a lovely little harbour. We enjoyed it. Then when the yacht was ready we set sail for the Humber to reach Grimsby docks.

The scenery on the way there was fantastic and we had no further problems. We sailed past the two forts which are on either side of the River Humber, then we had a slight mishap – we nearly got caught on a sandbank, but we managed to stay clear. We passed down the Humber and saw all the lights of Cleethorpes as we passed, because it was at night. It was like Christmas. Cleethorpes Promenade and Wonderland were lit up with many different-coloured lights. It was a wonderful sight.

We sailed through the lock gates and into Grimsby Dock Marina, where we tied up and spent time with our family before we sailed off up the east coast of Britain to reach Scotland.

When we set off it was a fine day. The sun was shining and the sea was flat calm. We put the sails out and made good progress. It was great. I was loving it. We were sailing along quite smoothly. Then after a day and night of sailing I felt terrible. I was sick and everything started spinning non-stop. I lay down in the cabin, but every time I tried to move everything was still spinning around at great speed. And I was vomiting. Then it started blowing a gale, which turned into a storm. I could not move, I was so sick. I lay watching Francis through the cabin window. He was trying to get the sails in, but he was being thrown about on the cabin roof. Then he managed it and tried getting the yacht under control. We were by now in a right storm and I could not help him. I could not move. I had to watch him doing everything on his own.

Then I heard him on the yacht radio saying, "This is Sea Flame Two. This is Sea Flame Two. [That was the name of our yacht.] I'm in trouble. I have both engines down. Sick wife on board. I need help."

I thought, 'Oh no, not again!'

He was telling them our position. They told him we were

close to Whitby, so the lifeboat would take us there and an ambulance would be waiting for us.

So we got towed in with paramedics seeing to me, and I was taken to Whitby Hospital because I had gone into panic. I couldn't breathe and I had to have oxygen and a drip. I was in there a few days as I was dehydrated. When I was well enough, Francis took me back on the yacht.

That was the second time we had been towed back to port by a lifeboat.

After Francis had had both of his engines reconditioned, and they had assured Francis they would be fine, we went on our way again. We had a great time, stopping at nearly every harbour on our way. I was sunbathing and getting quite a tan.

Sailing through the night we watched the lights on the shore, which were so scenic.

We did some fishing with our rods. The sea was good for us, like a millpond. I felt fit and healthy. Life was good – too good, because we hit trouble once again.

I was getting rather agitated with Francis, talking as if he was to blame, until he told me, "That's what you have to expect. That's the joy of sailing – rough seas and calm seas."

I said, "In that case, I don't like that kind of joy. I want you to take us into the nearest harbour until the sea is calm again."

We made sure we put our lifebelts on. The radio was warning every sailor the sea was changing into a force eight.

Francis said, "OK, we will run for the nearest port."

He checked his chart. The nearest was Hartlepool, so we headed for it. Then – just our luck! – both engines failed again and the sea struck us head-on. We couldn't turn out of it; we had to take the full force of it going over us. With no engines we could not turn around. We didn't even have time to shut the cabin door – the sea came over us, filling the cabin up. I was clinging on to the side of the cabin door. I was petrified. I thought, 'Try to keep calm – just don't go into panic again.' The sea kept going over us and each time I thought, 'Is this it? Will we be coming up again?'

Francis said, "Put this line on – it is secured to the yacht."

I said, "No, thank you. I don't want to go down with the yacht. I would sooner be free to take my chances swimming for it."

I was hanging on for dear life, but I noticed water running back into the sea. Every time it ran over us it ran away through the holes on the deck.

We had been swamped a few times and Francis had not had time to put a Mayday call out.

Francis said, "I'll cut the small lifeboat adrift and you hang on to the rope and jump in it."

But we must have had a guardian angel that day. I looked up and the lifeboat was alongside us. They had already slung a line, turned us round out of the waves and were towing us along with them, tied securely alongside their lifeboat. Our yacht could only do 4 mph with both engines going, but tied to the lifeboat we must have been doing two or three times that. We had never moved so fast, even with our sails out. I must say I have never felt so safe and happy as I was to see that lifeboat.

I said to myself, "I should have expected more trouble as they say it comes in threes."

They took us into Hartlepool and tied us up in the marina. The lifeboat crew told us we had been seen from the shore by one of the crew, and he knew we were in trouble as he could see us taking in the sea and not turning away from it. They said if we had been on any other yacht other than a catamaran we wouldn't have come back up; we would have gone down after getting swamped like that. We couldn't thank them enough for saving us and told them we did not even have time to send out a Mayday call, so we were very thankful we had been seen. The crewman told us he did not live far from the harbour and just happened to be looking out to sea with his binoculars.

Of course we hit the headlines once again. The people in the marina couldn't do enough for us – they were so kind and helpful, and even helped me to dry the yacht out and fetch us fresh water every day. Another couple of yacht owners helped

Francis to take both engines out. He had decided to buy two new engines as even he had had enough of the others failing him. The fishermen in the marina brought us a fry-up of fish every day. They gave us dry blankets, and a dry-cleaner's near the harbour let us take our clothes there and they washed and dried them for us. I had a free sauna every day, and chatted to the manageress who was in charge of it. She was so kind. She would come to our yacht every afternoon to take me for a sauna and a cup of tea.

Francis got his new engines in, sold the old ones and gave the proceeds to the lifeboat fund.

The yacht was all dried out and so were we. With all new utensils and new engines we were all ready for the off again after a month.

I loved Hartlepool and the people and was a bit scared about sailing again, but the other yacht owners said, "Well, your yacht brought you this far. We would love to have a catamaran – they are safer with the hazards of sailing and can take more of the sea than many other boats."

So I was talked round and decided to go, hoping this time it would be safe sailing. We sailed off, waving goodbye to all the good friends we had met, and carried on sailing up to Scotland.

We had no more trouble after that. Our new engines were great, which made me happy. Now we were living a fantastic life of sailing. Life was good, like Francis said it would be. We sailed into every harbour, staying at least a week in each one. I had never seen such pretty little harbours before.

We visited Scottish castles and lochs, passing islands in the sea – one full of gannets and one full of little puffins. We stopped to fish with our rods, catching fish for tea. We even had to send a diver down to cut away a lobster pot which had snagged on our propeller. He put the pot on our deck and in it were two lobsters, so we had them for tea. Seals were swimming round us on their backs with sea urchins balanced on their stomachs which they were trying to break open with a stone so that they could eat them. I was so happy. We enjoyed such scenic sights with sunshine all the way! We were both very brown and happy.

We reached Peterhead and tied up in the marina. We went visiting Francis's brothers and sisters and also his mother, who all lived in Scotland.

We went round Fife Castle – his mother lives near there. We went to Loch Lomond, then travelled through the Cairngorm Mountains, which were full of ice, snow and deer, saw waterfalls on the Isle of Skye, then visited Fort William and the site of the Battle of Culloden.

We had decided we wanted to settle down somewhere in Scotland, so we carried on sailing from Peterhead, going right round the north-east coast of Scotland, passing oil rigs and spotting dolphins, seals and basking sharks before sailing into Lossiemouth and getting a permanent berth for the yacht.

We bought a cottage called Denview in Slackhead, a couple of miles from Buckie, just a field away from the Moray Firth. There were nine cottages and our neighbours were all good people.

We settled down in our cottage and went travelling around Scotland. We visited the Black Isle Show in Inverness, and went ferry-hopping around the small isles and visited such places as Oban and Tobermory. We sailed mostly down the Moray Firth and in Spey Bay, along to Fraserburgh, down to Eyemouth, or right up to Dornoch and John o' Groats, visiting many more castles, lochs and forts.

I was on cloud nine, really enjoying my retirement. We had barbecues every Sunday with Francis's family. When they got together they would talk broad Scottish, and his mother would call me a foreigner. Francis's mother would bake oatcakes for half of the Fyvie villagers. It took me many years to understand what they were talking about. Whenever my family from Grimsby came up to see us, Francis's mother would tell all the village she had her family of foreigners coming up to see her. It was a twelve-hour run from where my family lived to reach us. They would make a holiday of it. And now I was a great-grandmother to three boys and a girl – with two of the boys being twins.

Francis's family would have clan meetings together. I would watch them dressed in their different tartans, playing bagpipes and drinking different whiskies.

When my family came up to see us we would take them on the yacht, fishing. They could not believe it when they caught four or more mackerel on one rod. We would catch so many that we would share them with our neighbours.

One of Francis's sisters lived in New Zealand and her daughter was getting married, so all the family that could make it would be going to the wedding. Francis and I went. It was to be a holiday for us: two weeks in New Zealand and two weeks in Australia, visiting a couple of his first cousins – a dream holiday for us. About thirty of the family went – nearly all the men in their kilts, including Francis. They had different clan kilts on, including Gordon Highlanders and Black Watch (which was Francis's).They all looked amazing, but we all had a good search by the airline when we landed – searching the Scottish uniforms – but because they were army kilts we got through.

In New Zealand we took up a full floor of the hotel, which was near the beach where the wedding would be. Francis and the men, especially the Scotsmen, were drinking whisky non-stop from landing until after the wedding. We women left them to it while we visited New Zealand, riding horses and swimming in hot streams.

Then Francis and I flew to Australia to see a couple of his cousins. One had a backpacking hotel, and it was so big it took up a full street. Of course, once again Francis was drinking whisky.

His cousin took us around Australia. We went on Bondi Beach. His cousin was swimming in the surf without any trouble, but they told us they had been swimming in it since they were children, when they had emigrated there. We went round New South Wales, visiting Sydney Harbour Bridge and seeing Sydney Opera House. We spent Australia Day there. Francis and I drove out to the bush, on the way visiting places that reminded us of *Crocodile Dundee*. Then we flew back home to Scotland, only stopping once to refuel the aeroplane.

When we arrived back in Aberdeen Airport it was back to reality. We were the last plane to land that day because the airport closed down due to the heavy snow and ice. We had to stay in B & Bs because we could not get to our home – the roads were closed.

After a couple of days we managed to follow a snowplough and managed to make it home. We were lucky our roof was still intact – most of Francis's brothers' roofs had fallen in. It had been snowing and freezing so many times that the roofs were falling in because of the heavy ice.

So after our dream holiday we were back home with a bang. We were iced up in our home with freezing snow and ice. Francis's family were used to it – they often got snowed in. With living in the Grampian Mountains, they never felt the cold.

We had lived in Scotland now for nine years and enjoyed every minute of it. Then his mother died. She had been a schoolteacher and worked in the church. I thought she was a lovely lady. She taught me how to speak Scottish – their kind – and when we went to visit her it was not a cup of tea and a biscuit, it was more a feast. It was no wonder I piled weight on. We went to a meeting of the clans in Shillingtor with Scottish dancing.

While going to his yacht one day Francis slipped on the slipway, knocking himself out by cracking his head on the ground. He never seemed to recover after that. Then he had a stroke which left him with three parts of his brain damaged, and although I loved living in Scotland, as it was such a beautiful scenic place, we sold up and moved to Grimsby to be near my family in case anything happened to me. In Scotland there would be no one to help me, as his family were spread around the wilds of Scotland. I was seventy and Francis nearly seventy-six. We bought a bungalow near my family.

Francis then had a second stroke – a major one this time – which paralysed his arm and one leg. Then he got blood clots on both lungs and various other ailments. It was touch and go for six months, on twenty-four-hour watch, but he pulled through. I had my husband back again – my companion and friend – I thought; but I soon found that yes, he was with me, but not in mind, only in body. He was in a wheelchair, and after all that he fell and smashed his ankle and had to have it reconstructed. So he was back in hospital having that fixed, so he could only walk a little way, which he does because he loves to potter around the garden. Now I was pushing around another husband in a wheelchair, only this time it would be harder because things were going to get even worse.

We don't realise what we have to lose in life, especially our health, until it happens to us. As I was going to find out, things were going to get so bad for me I would nearly give up trying; but you have to get on with life if not for yourself for your family, because they are precious. So I get on with life because life is also precious. So now I was going to find out how precious.

Francis was born in Scotland. He joined the army at the age of fifteen for twenty-five years. He was in the Royal Engineers and his trade was combat engineer 1, sheet metalworker 2. In the highest service examination he passed all the subjects. As a combat soldier he trained in wide-range construction and military engineering skills, including road and bridge construction, handling and use of explosives and operation of water-supply equipment. He had additional supervisory responsibilities and attained the rank of sergeant.

He was on Christmas Island, where he was one of the soldiers to watch H-bomb testing. He also went to Singapore, Thailand and Northern Ireland.

After leaving the army he worked as a prison officer in Rochester for fifteen years. While there he escorted many well-known murderers to court.

Part three relates how Francis and I deal and live with his dementia.

PART THREE

IN SICKNESS AND HEALTH

What it's like looking after a
husband who has dementia,
sickness and strokes?
Things he says and does
just one day in our life!

We were sat together silently
when suddenly he said to me,
"Where is she – where is my wife?"
I point at myself.
"I am your wife.
Look, look and see, it's me –
I am your wife."
He looks at me, his face so white.
"You are not my wife –
where is my wife?"

Prologue

I cannot believe I am now in my late seventies, but I am.
Although everyone I know tells me I look years younger, I
think to myself, 'They are only being polite.' Because let
alone being seventy-five, I feel like I am ninety when I get
up in the morning and my aches and pains start. It's then I tell
myself I am about ready for the knacker's yard and it is about
time I was given the needle. That's what my first husband
used to say to me when his bones started creaking and he

started coughing – he died of lung cancer aged sixty-two. Now my second husband, who is eighty, has every ailment going for him, plus having had two strokes, two lungs full of blood clots, prostate trouble (which makes him go to the toilet every hour of the day and night), high blood pressure, diabetes, high cholesterol and, as if that is not enough, one of his strokes left him with his left arm and leg paralysed. And, to put the icing on the cake, he always falls because he can only walk ten yards before he loses his balance – which one day he did, smashing his ankle to pieces. They fixed it together as best as they could, but now it is badly deformed so that his foot drags along the ground.

So now it's my turn. I tell him he's ready for the knacker's yard and he should be given the needle. It's a good job he knows I am joking and we can both have a good laugh.

He tells everybody he is thirty – sometimes he will say forty. He really does believe he is. Two years after his last stroke we found out he had dementia, so now he is in a wheelchair. It has to be a hand-pushed one. He cannot have a mobility one because he does not remember where he lives or where he's going – he gets lost – so I have to push him everywhere.

I am his one and only full-time carer, his lifeline, his wife of thirteen years. I know nothing about medicine or nursing, so I have been pushed in at the deep end in caring for him. I have to give him so many tablets and I have to work them out by the hours in the day. One lot of his tablets is warfarin, which I understand is rat poison. It is an anticoagulant, to prevent blood clots in his lungs – it is to thin his blood. We have a good laugh about this. I tell him even rat poison cannot kill him off. Every week he has to have INR jabs.

So now my days and nights are worked out for me. I have to take him to so many appointments – hospitals, clinics and doctors – for all his different ailments besides caring for his needs. Apart from that I am now head of the house, having to do everything a man of the house would do, like mending things around the home, paying bills and mowing the lawn, as well as my own work, including washing, cleaning, cooking and shopping. I would sooner bring another ten children up. Sometimes I tell myself I wish I was the one being looked after. I would have no worries, no stress and no hard work. I'd be getting fed, clothed, taken out on holidays – I would have some rest. I would be living in a world without a care, everything done for me – paradise. I tell myself his world is far better than mine and this was not what I signed up for, but after some mind-searching I have to admit to myself, "Oh, yes, I did sign up for it!" Because what did I say when I married him in church before God? "In sickness and in health, for better or worse. . . ." So here I am now, living it – his sickness. I felt guilty for thinking I should not be looking after him, and I felt guilty for having the weakness to feel sorry for myself. I felt ashamed. I told myself, "He has looked after and cared about me for the last sixteen years. So now the tide has turned, and now it is my time to do the caring. It's payback time. Be strong and stop feeling sorry for yourself. Get on with it."

I remember what my mother would always say to me: "You made your bed, now lie in it."

Francis never needs much sleep and I cannot say that surprises me, because every couple of hours in the day he falls asleep for at least ten minutes at a time. When I tell him to try not to go to sleep so many times in the day he tells me he has not been to sleep, he was only resting his eyes. It's the same old story every time. When he nods off in front of the great-grand-babies they point and giggle at him, telling me to look at great-grandad because he has fallen asleep and is snoring with his mouth open, catching flies. It tickles them. They stand there with their little hands over their mouths, looking up towards the ceiling, trying not to laugh.

Then when he opens his eyes they tell him, "Grandad, you were fast sleep with your mouth open and snoring!"

He says, "I was not – I was only pretending."

They tell him, "You were so sleeping, Grandad. Pull our legs – they have bells on."

He needs constant care, so I never get much sleep – only snatches when I can, because I have to watch him every time he gets out of bed in case he loses his balance and falls. Sometimes I think I could sleep for a full month if I got the chance.

I get a good laugh out of him when he tries to dress himself without my help. He stands there struggling for some time, getting angry with himself because he cannot manage it on his own and he is too proud to ask for my help. When he has finished trying and has tied himself in knots, then he will let me help him. Then I have to try to unravel him. Everything he has tried to put on will be inside out. His underpants will be down around his ankles with his trousers pulled up over the top of them, but they won't be pulled up enough to cover his bum. His sweatshirt will be stuck in layers around his neck, strangling his neck, and both hands will be entwined in it so he cannot move. He stands there until his face goes red and he reluctantly lets me help him. I have a job getting him unravelled myself. Then, after I have got him undressed and dressed again, he will try to tie a bow in his belt cord. He will try for some time until he gets frustrated and gives up. Then because he has not been able to fasten it himself he drops his hands to his sides and thumps them on his legs. Then he starts jumping up and down, throwing his hands in the air as far as he can get them up, just like a spoilt child. For me to see him this way, struggling along, trying to dress on his own, not being able to do the smallest things for himself that were so easy for him before is so trying for me. It upsets me sometimes. I get so annoyed, but I have to remind myself that he is a very sick man and is only trying his best to remain the man he used to be. I tell myself that he is very lucky to still be alive after going through what he went through with all his sicknesses. But I do tell myself it should be me who is jumping up and down with the frustration and stress after the hard work of looking after him the way I have to. I deserve a medal for what I have to go through.

It does distress me and upset me. It was only a few years ago that he was a strong and healthy man, so full of energy.

We both would go walking every day and swimming twice a week. Being a Scotsman, he would do Scottish dancing.

He had a yacht – a catamaran. He was a great skipper, a great sailor. He would take our family out on it, fishing some days, sailing other days. The children could not believe it when they caught four fish on one rod. When he took them fishing he knew just where to take them to catch the fish, which was just off Lossiemouth, Scotland. But now he can hardly do anything for himself.

His first stroke was in 2010. It damaged his brain in three parts, which caused his dementia, but at the time we did not know this. His next stroke, three years later, was a major one. It confined him to a wheelchair and it was still two years after this that a doctor who treats mental illness diagnosed he had vascular dementia. Over the last four years previous to finding this out I knew something was wrong with him. At first he was forgetting things, but we would both make excuses, covering it up. Neither of us would admit anything was wrong with him. He was so fit, still doing his fishing and sailing, but covering up a lot of mistakes he made, until one day he came home after supposedly checking everything on his yacht was in working order – something he did once a week.

This day the electrician came home with him. He took me to one side. He said to me, "Are you aware of your husband's mental state? I think there is something wrong because I have had to mend the lights on the yacht three times in the last month and every time I have replaced the wires he has pulled them out again, causing a fire on the yacht. I really do believe there is something wrong with his mind."

Of course he told me this while my husband was busy outside so he could not hear what we were discussing.

I told him, "Yes, I was thinking along the same lines." I told him Francis had been mending things that were not broken, I told him he was forgetting important things and covering up his actions. We both agreed. We thought it was brain trouble from his stroke, so the electrician said he would mend the lights again so that I could sell the yacht, because it would be a great shame to just let him carry on destroying it. So that's what we did.

We had moved back to live in Grimsby to be near my family because I knew things would get a lot worse, which they did after his second stroke – a major one. He got really bad. He was forgetting his family and where he lived for months at a time. Memories would come back to him for a while, then he would forget them again. I would repeat myself over and over, telling him about his family. He would say, "Oh, yes, I remember!" But when I asked him just two minutes later he had forgotten again. I had to keep telling him where he lived and how old he was, but it was a waste of time on my part so I made sure he always had his name and address in his wallet at all times for safety.

I put photographs all over the house of me and him and our children. He points at them and always asks me who they are. When I have told him he will say, "Oh, yes, I remember." But I can see by his face that he doesn't. It hurts me to see that he does not know his own family. It comes to him sometimes, but does not stay for long. I tell myself it's not his fault, it's the sickness, but it still breaks my heart. I feel so sad for him because I know he has no memories that he can think back on.

When I take him out for the day he will be happy and contented. He will say to me, "I have enjoyed my day out – it was great."

I ask him, "Where was it that we went?"

He sits thinking about it for a while, then says, "I don't know. I cannot think where I have been."

He always says he is thirty. Sometimes I burst his bubble: I say, "You wish, but I'm afraid you are eighty!"

He looks so shocked and amazed, saying, "Never! I never am!"

I give him a pen and paper. I write down what year he was born and I write down what year we are in, then I tell him to write the years in between. He begins writing things down, and he looks like he is working it out.

I think, 'Good – he is thinking things out. It will do him good to train his brain.'

After quite a while I say, "Have you worked it out, then?"

He says, "Yes, I am thirty."

I look at what he has written down. It is a load of scribble. I just pass it by. I tell myself he is happy thinking he is half his age so I should leave it be. It certainly works for him, but it would not work for me. I could not tell myself I'm years younger and try to believe it – I look in the mirror and it brings me back to reality.

Sometimes I find him sat in the living room in the middle of the night, in the dark. He's looking around the room with a distant look on his face. I can see he is wondering where he is and he looks frightened.

I think to myself, 'What a cruel illness dementia is, especially when you have to watch it happening day and night to someone who is close to you.' I always feel so sorry for him.

I take hold of his hand and I say, "What's up, then?"

One one occasion he said, "Where are the children? Where have they gone?"

And I knew then he had drifted back in time to when his children were small, at least fifty years ago.

I smiled at him, trying to reassure him, saying, "Don't you remember? The children are all grown up now. They have children of their own – you are a great-grandad now."

I showed him photographs, telling him who everyone was.

He said, "Oh, yes, I remember." But I could see by his face that he did not.

I took him to bed, telling him we would visit the children tomorrow, and he settled for that and got back into bed; but he was in and out of bed all night, and I could see by his face that he was wondering where he was.

I had a walk-in bath fitted with a hydrotherapy spa and fitted seat with a shower right above his head. He loves it and so do I. He only has one a week because he has a weak heart valve and it tires him out, but he always tells me it makes him feel good. It is also good for his circulation – when he has a bad day and cannot move or bend his knees I give him the hydrotherapy bath and he can bend his knees again.

It is also a godsend for me. My knees have to be replaced at some time in the future, because of wear and tear on them, and at times I get a lot of pain from them. At one time I was given painkilling tablets, but I was on them for so long I ended up in hospital twice with internal bleeding, so now I cannot take painkilling tablets. Instead my doctor gives me painkilling injections in both knees every six months and I am practically pain-free. Those injections are a godsend for me. In fact, until I have my knee replacements they are a lifeline for me.

I rarely have time to even think about or complain about my ailments because I am busy trying to keep up with his, so when he starts moaning to me about his aches and pains I remind him that in this world there are so many people a lot worse off than the two of us; we have a lot to be thankful for.

We have each other to moan to, and we have a good family who are always willing to help whenever we let them. We take each day as it comes, and if it's a good day I am very thankful and happy for it; if it's a bad day I still try to be happy and kind and loving for him.

I never plan anything ahead because with his sickness we never know what is coming next, so tomorrow takes care of itself. I don't worry about what all our tomorrows may bring – we both deal with whatever is going to be when it comes along, which is sometimes worse with each passing day. But, no matter what, I make sure he wants for nothing, even though sometimes it drains me of energy and patience. At least I can remember all the good times we both had together, which is more than I can say for Francis. He has no memories whatsoever.

He always made sure I wanted for nothing. He took me halfway round the world on wonderful holidays, and we would go cycling nearly every day. Now, because of his broken ankle, he cannot push the pedals round and, with him always losing his balance, he cannot even walk on the beach – sand makes him fall over.

All of those things we did together he cannot do any more. They are no longer there for us. None of us realise what we have to lose until it becomes no longer feasible. We never know what is around the corner, what lies in wait, until what we have is taken away from us and we are unable to get it back. We never realise how much those precious little things mean to us.

I thank the Lord I can still remember, and that's a wonder because Francis messes with my brain. I tell myself it's a wonder that I still have my marbles, because he will say to me, "It is Friday today, is it not?"

And I will put him right, telling him, "No, it is Monday!"

But he carries on saying it over and over again, and I keep on trying to put him right until I feel like a parrot, always repeating myself. Then I tell myself it is no good trying to make him know that he is wrong, because of his sickness it just does not go in. He cannot grasp it. Then I give in to him just to shut him up.

I say, "OK, it is Friday today."

But by then he has brainwashed me by repeating it so many times and I begin to doubt myself. I have to check the calendar to make sure I have got it right, and even then I have a final look at the newspaper to make sure. So now I don't try to put him right because I will be wasting my time. I cannot help his sick brain.

One morning after breakfast he put his hat on his head, picked up his walking stick, put his glasses on (which he only uses for reading) and, still in his nightwear with his slippers on, said to me, "Come on, then, it's time to go."

I asked him, "Where are you wanting to go?"

He replied, "We have to go to hospital."

I asked him, "Are you sick?"

He said, "No, but I have to see the nurse today."

I thought I must have forgotten one of his appointments, so I checked. I had not. So I explained to him, "We don't have to see the nurse today." And I had to show him the appointment book to calm him down. I told him, "We can take a rest from going to the nurse for at least a week."

He said, "Oh, that's good. Thank goodness for that."

He took his hat and glasses off and sat down to rest, but two minutes later he did the same thing again.

I thought to myself, 'I'm not going to keep on repeating myself to him.' So I just carried on ignoring him and getting on with my work, making sure that the key was not in the door so he could not go out. In the end he sat reading.

I found him sat on his chair in the middle of the night in the dark, like I have so many times before. I turned on the light. He was staring around. I could see by his face that he was confused.

He looked at me and said, "Who are you?"

I could see he did not know me. I felt like I had been hit with a hammer – that really hurt me. I started crying in front of him. I tried not to, but could not help it. After all we had gone through I never thought he would forget me.

I said to him, "I am your wife."

He said, "You are not my wife."

I asked him, "Who am I, then?"

He replied, "I do not know." And then he started crying, holding his head. He said pleadingly to me, "I have to go, don't I? I don't want to, but I have to, don't I?"

I took his hand and told him, "You don't have to go anywhere. This is your home and I am your wife."

I showed him photographs of our wedding day.

He looked so relieved and started smiling, saying, "Oh, thank goodness, that is me and you."

He went to bed and slept.

In the morning I took him out in his wheelchair to the church where we were married, showing him and telling him that was where we got wed.

He said, "Oh, yes, but who are you?"

Then I knew I was wasting my time again. I could not even get him to remember me, his own wife of thirteen years. How could he forget me? I knew that there was no way he would ever forget me if it was not for his sickness. I just had to wait for his memory to return, whenever, hoping and praying it would not take long.

I asked myself, "What if he never remembers me again?"

I woke at 5 a.m. to the sound of running water. I thought, 'Oh, no, not again.' I knew it was him. I found him in the bathroom – he was having a shower with his nightwear on. He was stood in the bath. He had left the door open and put the plug in, so with the shower on the water was running out of the bath into the hallway and living room. I pulled the plug out, turned the shower off, took his wet clothes off, dried and dressed him, then made him sit and read so that I could mop everything up, all before breakfast.

When I had done everything he said to me, "I had a good shower. I am refreshed."

I said, "Oh, good for you. I am very pleased about that, but next time you want a shower wait for me so that I can help. You should not shower by yourself. Because of your sickness you might fall. And you have flooded the hallway out again."

He said he was sorry and would wait for my help next time, but I knew he wouldn't because two minutes after I have asked him to do something he has forgotten it.

After breakfast one day he was getting so agitated and I could not calm him, so I took him out and pushed him around town in his wheelchair. People who know him will stop and talk to him. They always say, "You look so fit and well." And he does, even though he is still a very sick man. But I, his carer, am looking knackered and worn out even though one of my daughters often comes to give me a break.

One time I felt like catching a train, or even an aeroplane, to get away from it all – as far away as possible – and telling no one, but then I thought of my family. It would hurt them and upset them not knowing where I was, thinking and worrying about me, not knowing if I was dead or alive. I thought about what my mother would say to me: "Stop feeling sorry for yourself. You made your bed, now lie in it."

I tell myself, "What must he be feeling himself?"

Once again I think, 'Stop feeling sorry for yourself. Get on with whatever life throws at you.' And I hate myself. How could I think of running away from a bit of hard work? Running away from a sick husband! I would feel ashamed of myself. It is not as if I need any other life than the one I already have. After I have told myself all this I have got it out of my system and I feel happier and a lot better for it. I feel I can face anything that comes my way. Then I spoil him as much as I can. I take him round the town, shopping and to a good carvery for his dinner, because he likes me pushing him about.

We were sat in the doctor's waiting room waiting to see the nurse for his usual INR jab, which he has weekly. We both sat watching the screen, waiting for his name to come up. It was warning hay fever sufferers there was going to be a lot of pollen around because of the heat and telling them that they had to be careful.

He said to me, "I want some of that pollen."

I told him, "Oh no, you can forget about wanting pollen. You have enough on your plate to be going on with with all your ailments. We can do without any more, so forget it."

He was getting quite annoyed with me, saying, "I want some pollen. Get me some or I will get some myself."

Everyone was laughing at him.

I tried calming him down, explaining to him, telling him why he should not want any. I told him, "You cannot buy pollen – it comes from flowers because of the heat, and if you breathe it in it will make you cough and sneeze, make you poorly and full of cold, and your eyes will run." I felt like I was explaining it to a child.

All the while we were waiting to see the nurse, he still kept asking for some pollen.

A SYMBOL OF OUR LOVE

You gave to me a red, red rose,
Telling me your love was true.
I told you I was true to you.
I watered it from day to day
Until it started to wilt away.
I could not let my pretty rose fade
After the commitments we had made –
It was a symbol of our love.

I pressed it in my little book
So I could always take a look.
That red, red rose you gave to me
Is always there for me to see.
My very first rose is there to stay;
I could never throw that rose away –
It was a symbol of our love.

Every day I open my book –
Every day I have a look –
Bringing back memories of you and me,
Reminding me of what used to be.
That red red rose I took from you,
That rose will always see me through –
It was a symbol of our love.

You gave to me a red, red rose,
Telling me your love was true.
I told you I was true to you.
I watered it from day to day
Until it started to wilt away.
I could not let my pretty rose fade
After the commitments we have made –
It was a symbol of our love.

I always have a vase of imitation flowers in the living room because they never die.

On many occasions Francis says to me, "Them flowers are pretty, but if you don't keep water in the vase they will die."

I try telling him they are fake flowers, but he cannot distinguish the difference between imitation and live flowers. He keeps trying to water them, and when I tell him they do not need water he looks at me as if I am stupid and he gets angry with me, saying that I am leaving them to die. So to shut him up I have to put water in the vase.

He has done it again! He managed to get himself another ailment: a problem with his bladder. So there is another hospital trip every six months to see how he is getting along. They have put him on a trial drug and I have to keep a check on what drink goes in and what comes out. I ought to get a job as a nurse with the things I have had to do for him, treating all his different ailments and giving him his different tablets. At least he does not have a catheter fitted, because he had one before and he kept pulling it out. The tablets did the trick.

We had a gas cooker in our kitchen. He would turn the knobs on, but he could not light the gas. I had to have it taken out and replace it with an electric one for safety reasons. That was only one of the adjustments I had to make around the place to make things easier and safer for him, including having handrails fitted inside and outside.

I am pleased he can walk a couple of yards, so he can go to the bathroom. Even so, when he is having a bad week I have to help him as he loses his balance a lot.

I'm glad his wheelchair folds up and fits in the car so I can take him out. Sometimes even that is a hard job, trying to push him through some of our streets. The holes in some pavements make it hard as the small front wheels catch in them, bringing us to a full stop and jarring the handles into my chest. The fact that he is a heavy man does not help either. I keep telling him I should put him on a diet, but he just laughs. I tell him I am running out of puff.

He says, "You are not starving me. I like food!"

And he certainly does.

I'm so lucky to have such a good family who help whenever they can. My eldest daughter takes us with her for a weekend break and when we go out on excursions she will take over pushing him around in his wheelchair. That's when I feel freedom. It might not sound much, but for me it is paradise for a while. It is like taking a weight off my shoulders. It gives me the chance to relax. Apart from that, I have no meals to cook and every night there is entertainment in the hotel. A long weekend of freedom! Plus we are driven home the scenic way, straight to our door. It is a full weekend of heaven – no responsibilities for me.

One beautiful day I took him to the park for fresh air and peace and quiet to relax and feed the ducks. Because he had had me up most of the night, running after him for one thing and another, it would do us both some good and maybe settle him down – or so I thought! I was pushing him around the flower beds, enjoying the peacefulness, when a couple of dogs came bounding up to us not on their leads. They started barking and snarling around him in his wheelchair, while the owners were having a job trying to get them under control. I pushed him away from them as I could see he was getting upset and uneasy and I was also frightened of them. We got away from them and went to the café for a cup of tea and a toasted teacake – which we always have when we go to the park.

We had just got settled and were enjoying our cuppa when in came two young girls. They started running around the tables and chairs, pushing into anyone who was in the way, shouting and screaming at each other.

So I got him out of the way and took him to the pond to feed the ducks. We were throwing them the bread and, lo and behold, the ducks were fighting each other for it. Then a load of seagulls and pigeons started swooping down on the ducks, pulling the bread from out of their beaks. And, to top it all off, the fish were popping up from underneath for the bread, so the poor ducks were getting assailed from above and below. They had had enough and went away, quacking as they left.

They weren't the only ones who had had enough – so had we. I pushed Francis back to the car and we went home. I thought to myself, 'What's up with everybody today? It must be the heat!' We got more peace and quiet at home.

One morning I was waiting for him to get up for his breakfast, which I had already made, but he was making no move to get out of bed.

I said, "OK, come on."

He pulled himself up into a sitting position and said, "I am not getting up today. My legs are so heavy – they feel like lead and are so stiff. I cannot walk."

I had to force him out by telling him, "Look, you have to get up and walk as I'm not strong enough to lift you up and push you around in your wheelchair inside the house as well as outside. Come on, you have to force yourself like I have to on many a day to look after you, and me with my bad knees. I don't give in, so neither should you. No matter how hard it is, you must never give in."

He got out of bed, but not without a lot of struggling and moaning. I thought to myself, 'Thank goodness it worked this time.' I shamed him into getting out of bed.

After his breakfast I helped him to do his exercises, like his therapist showed him, moving his legs up and down. After that he did his walk up the drive a couple of times. I don't usually have to force him out of bed or practically force him to do his walks as he normally does them on his own, but now and again he will try his best to stay in bed – especially on his bad days, when he feels down and listless. I know I must not give in to him because I know he will take to his bed soon enough one day.

One morning he told me, "I cannot have my walk today because it is raining."

I told him, "That is no excuse, but you must not forget your cap because if the rain falls on your head it will make your hair grow."

He looked quite pleased with himself and said, "Will it? Will it make my hair grow on top of my head?"

I said, "Yes, so make sure you put your hat on because you have enough hair for the hairdresser to cut already. And make sure you don't slip."

He said, "Well, I'd better go for my walk now."

He went out minus his hat and he had a spring in his step.

I noticed when he came back in he looked in the mirror and was running his fingers through the couple of hairs that he had on top of his head, touching them and pulling them up. I could see he was looking to see if any hair had grown.

I thought to myself, 'Some men are more vain than some women, and even at his age he is one of them.'

He did not forget that in a hurry – he went out in the rain a few times after that without his hat on.

Why he should bother at his age if he has hair or not, and with all his ailments and suffering, I don't know. But at least I had found a way once again to get him to not think twice about doing his walk, especially in the rain. Whatever makes him happy!

We went for a day out to a zoo near Devon. It was at least fifty acres. It was fantastic, full of so many amazing animals and other wildlife. They supplied mobility scooters. I thought it a long way to push him around in his wheelchair, so he had a go on one and did quite well. So I let him have one. They only go at about 4 mph and he couldn't go outside so I thought it would be all right – we could keep an eye on him and stay with him, and also he was having a good few days with memory so off we went. There was delight in his eyes, and he was showing off and proud of himself because he was in control. He was driving up and down the hills, smiling and grinning away to himself, always leaving me behind. I had a hard job keeping up with him. I was running and puffing and panting, trying to keep up with him, worrying in case he got lost.

He made sure he did not miss one bird or animal. He was laughing at me trying my best to keep up with him. I kept telling him to slow down and wait for me or else I was going to take the scooter off him. Jokingly I thought to myself, 'I should have used my brain like I am always telling him to do. I should have got one for myself, but it's too late to think about that now.'

After running after him up and down those hills at that zoo I was shattered. I must have lost a few pounds in weight for my pains, but at least he had a fantastic time before I told him to pay the bill. He spent at least ten minutes trying to get his wallet out of his pocket. He was pulling and struggling.

Everyone was laughing because I said, "What's up? Have you stuck it in there again with glue like you always do when I ask you to pay, hoping I will get fed up with waiting and pay it myself." But this time, after all the running after him, I was determined he should pay. I said, "Let me help you get it out."

And I did! It was out in a flash and he paid for once!

Most days when I push him through the town in his wheelchair he insists on taking his walking stick with him. I have to let him because he needs it when he gets out of the chair to go to the toilet. If it wasn't for that I would make him leave it behind, because while I am pushing him along he indicates with his stick which way he thinks I am going. When I go left he points it that way, waving the stick up and down, then does the same when we go right. If we don't turn he holds the stick straight up in the air, pointing it front and back. It does not matter who is in the way, they get a whack with it. I have had a few on my head. I end up taking it off him, and that is hard to do because he will try hanging on to it for as long as he can. I have to explain he cannot keep whacking people with it, because one of them will be taking it off him and whacking him back one day. He still grins and tries to keep it until I get mad with him, telling him to behave himself and give it to me or else I shall push him and his chair up the highest hill, tie him in and let it go. That does it – I think he believes me. He lets me have the stick reluctantly, so then I end up having to carry it.

I have to deal with his behaviour in the way you might deal with children. I cannot put him on the naughty step, so have to threaten him in another way.

One of his sisters came for a couple of days to see him and to see how he was getting on. She makes the journey a couple of times a year. She travels by train as she lives in Scotland, so we always meet her at the station.

He needs most of my attention, but she is his sister and she must worry for him; so I have to get on with it even though I could do without the extra work. With him I am at it day and night, but I understand her concern for her brother.

As soon as he saw her outside he recognised her at once. He smiled and waved to her. That made her happy because the last time she came he did not show recognition all the time she was here – he kept asking me who she was. She understands that he does not remember even family sometimes – that's the way dementia goes. So she was happy and so was he.

It does him good to see his family and it is generally not possible to travel to see them because they live so far away. He needs constantly looking after, so I cannot travel far with him.

She rested the first day because of all the travelling she did to get here. The next day we took her to The Deep, in Hull. They both enjoyed watching the fish and penguins. Francis thought they were cute.

The next day he was feeling fit and happy, so I took the pair of them to Cleethorpes. They had a good play on the slot machines – he enjoyed putting his money in, if he won anything or not. Then we pushed him along some of the seafront, watching some trawlers and yachts come up the River Humber from the North Sea between the two forts on the river.

The next day we all went to the Fishing Heritage Centre so she could see a trawler iced up and see how the fishermen caught their fish and how the skipper's cabin used to be and what they dressed in while at sea. The pair of them thought it quite interesting.

Then it was time for her to catch a train for home, but before she went she said to me not to expect too much from him; he would get worse.

I told her, "Yes, I know, and I will deal with it as it comes along."

She told me I am an angel the way I care and look after him.

I told her, "No, I am no angel. I feel guilty sometimes because I let him annoy me and stress me out, and I should not because he tries his best when he can."

She told me, "Don't ever feel guilty about getting stressed. Everyone does, but it's how you deal with it that counts. And I see you deal with it quite well."

Those few words took a heavy burden off my mind, because I did not know if I was caring for him like I should. It took the guilt feeling away, knowing I was doing right for him and looking after him properly. Those words made me know I was doing the best I could, and he would not be looked after any better than he was being looked after now. I felt a lot happier about myself.

We left her at the station, where she said goodbye to us.

On the way home Francis said to me, "Who was that we were on holiday with?"

So I told him, "That was your sister."

He said, "Oh, yes, I remember."

I could see by his face he could not, but at least he had had a good time. It was back down to earth with a bang.

One morning I looked at his face and one of his eyes was full of blood. I thought, 'Here we go again – another ailment.' I was hoping it would be another busted vein, which he has had before – a small one that soon clears up. But no, we were not so lucky this time. With him being on warfarin it was a bleed in his eye, and it took a year of going backwards and forwards to the specialist at the hospital for laser treatment before it got better.

It's hard work caring for him day and night with his dementia and all these ailments and hospital visits. It really is very hard because as soon as one thing clears up another ailment takes its place.

Francis enjoys his trips to the nurse, hospitals and clinics. He thinks he's on holiday, so at least he gets enjoyment out of the trips.

When he gets a pain he never tells me. I have to look for the signs. He will hold or rub the place where he is in pain. If he does that a couple of times in a day I will know he has a pain; if he keeps it up all day and into the next then I take him to see his doctor, because he cannot explain to me how bad it is or what it is.

One day he sat watching me doing some gardening, then I saw him go into the garage. After a while I went to check on him, he was busy mending an old rake that the end had fallen off. I could see that he wasn't doing anything to hurt himself, so I left him to it and carried on with my gardening. A while later he came up to me with the rake, showing me what he had done. I examined it and saw that he had made a good job of screwing the rake back on, so I told him how pleased I was with him and said he had done a good job for me. He went back into the garage with a big smile on his face, feeling quite happy because he had done something useful. So I left him to it and went in to cook the dinner, saying to myself, "He cannot come to any harm in the garage as there are only a few tools in there. He will be pottering about, trying to mend things and feeling good with himself."

When dinner was done I went to fetch him. He was stood with a screwdriver trying to unscrew the plug on the wall with the electric turned on, and he had strung loads of electric wire across the beams of the garage. I grabbed the screwdriver off him. He did not want me to have it. He was fighting me to keep hold of it. I turned the electric off at the mains. He kept telling me he would mend the plugs as they were loose. I told him he must never try mending plugs again because he would electrocute himself and me and that the electrician – a special man – was the only one who could touch plugs; even I could not. I felt like I was telling a child off for being naughty. I told him he could mend the rakes and brushes for me, but I must be with him when he does. He was happy with that and I took him for his dinner.

I locked the garage and hid the key – so that was another key to hide alongside many others, for his safety and mine.

I knew in the back of my mind I should never have trusted him in there on his own in the first place, but these things he does shows me dangers are everywhere with a person who has dementia because they cannot see danger.

In his younger days he was a sergeant in the army dishing out orders, and the habit has never left him. He tries dishing them out to me – fetch me this, pass me that, do this, do that. I do it sometimes without thinking, then I stop and think to myself, 'I am not his dog – I have to do enough for him as it is.'

So I stand there and give him a salute, saying, "Yes sir, no sir, three bags full, sir!" and "What did your last slave die of? Was it hard work? Did you work them to death like you try to do to me?" Then I tell him, "While you can still walk, get off your backside and do it yourself, even if you have to drag yourself around."

He will always say sorry, and he will do it himself even though it takes him a long time.

If he's trying to dress himself I watch him struggle, but he manages it in the end. Then I will help put him right, because his trousers might be back to front and his shirt buttons in the wrong holes; he might have put on different-colour socks and his shoe backs might be trodden down with putting them on without undoing them. But I don't mind. While he is dressing himself – or should I say trying to? – it is keeping him active and keeping him moving around, stopping his muscles seizing up.

I have to keep him going because if he had his way he would let me do all his running around, and that means he would give in and take to his bed a lot quicker, but he does only try it on his bad days. On a good day he tries to do everything himself without me asking him. I watch him and leave him to it. What is that old saying? 'You have to be cruel to be kind.'

Sometimes I watch him while he is reading. He sits up straight with both arms outstretched holding his book open, supposedly still reading, but he is fast asleep, not moving a muscle. Anyone else would have dropped the book or put their arms down once they had fallen asleep, but not him. He will stay in that position for at least an hour without moving, snoring with his mouth open. Then when he wakes up he just carries on reading.

I said to him one day, "Oh, you are awake! Did you have a good sleep, then?"

He denied being asleep – he told me he was just resting his eyes.

"So you can read your book with your eyes closed, snoring away, not moving, staying in one position? I bet it boils down to when you were a young boy soldier on guard duty, falling asleep resting on your gun too tired to stay awake but not daring to move so no one would know, because if you were caught you would be shot."

He said, "Who, me? Never! Let me tell you I was dedicated to doing my very best to be a good soldier, to be a man and train well."

I said, "Yes, I can see that you trained yourself all right, on how to sleep well while on guard!"

He just laughed it off.

We got a nice surprise from one of the diabetic nurses one day. He had been a borderline diabetic for eight years, controlling it by diet. She told us he is a pre-diabetic from now on, as his levels have been good for the last two years. That meant fewer clinic appointments and check-ups for him, lightening my load – less work for me; one less ailment for him.

We were both happy about that, but I could not help thinking to myself, 'It will not be long before something else takes its place.' And it did!

While seeing the surgeon at the hospital for one of his appointments, which he has plenty of, the surgeon told me Francis had quite a lot of kidney stones. He showed me his X-rays. I could not believe it – there were four on one side and three on the other side, one of which was a big one. But, with all his other ailments, it could wait until they had to be removed.

I could not help thinking to myself, 'So, more trips to the hospital for him so they can keep an eye on his stones!'

These surgeons and doctors do a wonderful job of taking care of their patients' well-being – especially Francis's! The ailments they have put right for him, never giving up on him! I admire all of them, especially as he is eighty years old and, in my mind, on his way out. But no, they carry on regardless. I tell him he is a very lucky man and well looked after by everyone. I call him the walking wounded, or walking dead. I tell him I think of him as a zombie. We have a good laugh about this – even he admits that is what he is.

He called me by my name one day. I was wondering if I had heard him rightly, because it was the first time he had remembered my name for the last six months. It made me feel good for a while, but I told myself, "I wonder how long he will remember me for this time?" His memory takes longer to come back to him each time he loses it. One day it will be gone forever – he won't get it back. I just cannot figure dementia out. I will never understand it. I tell myself, "How can he remember family and friends one day and forget everything and everyone the very next day?"

One day he can work something out; another day he cannot even work out the simplest of things. I call them good days and bad days. On good days his mind is there, and on bad days his mind is gone.

On one of his good days we were sat watching a quiz show. I could not believe it – he was shouting the answers out and getting them right.

I told him, "You're brainy today!"

185

Even I did not know the answers.

He laughed and smiled and I could see he was very proud of himself. He even followed me into the garden and he was stretching up and bending down, pulling up weeds, leaning on his stick. Even his balance was good.

Looking at him and listening to him, no one would have believed there was anything much wrong with him, but then another day he will be quite different. On his bad days I have to just about force him out of his bed. He will lie there saying he cannot walk, he cannot bend his knees, his legs feel like lead. When I finally get him out of the bed I have to help him bathe and dress. If I leave him to try to dress himself it takes so long, and then I have to dress him in the end because he ties himself in knots.

I have to force him to walk a couple of yards with my help; otherwise he would stay confined to his chair. When I take him out in his wheelchair I have to practically lift him in and out of it, and on bad days I even have to be with him when he goes to the bathroom to make sure he does not fall.

Sometimes he has confusing days. He will sit there staring around, and I can see by his face he is trying to remember something. I can see he is feeling worried.

Then he will say to me, "Where is my pension book? I must go to the post office and get my pension."

Then I have to explain to him, like I have so many times before, "You are a pensioner now – you don't have a book. The army pension goes into your bank and they pay all your bills for you because you don't remember your number."

I show him a statement, and that makes him happy until the next time he asks about it. Then he will blame it on me, saying, "I wish you would tell me these things, because it is the first time I have heard about it."

I tell him, "I will show you your statement every month, then, from now on." And that satisfies him until the next time.

I get a bit fed up with having to explain these things to him, but it is the only way I can calm him down about his pension. I tell myself it is because he is worried he is not earning his keep. I tell him he has no need to worry about anything like that because his memory loss is because of his sickness, and all he needs to worry about is getting better.

He always gives a big sigh of relief and says to me, "Oh, that's good. Thank you for telling me. I don't remember being sick or being in hospital."

I tell him he was in for nearly six months with one thing and another, but he won't believe me. He always says, "Never! Not me."

So I tell him, "Well, it is best forgotten."

One day he was stood in the hallway looking quite dazed, staring around and even looking at the ceiling. He stayed there looking for a while until I asked him what was up.

He said, "I don't know – I have forgotten what I was doing. I don't remember where I was going. I don't know where I am."

I said to him, "Don't worry – you are at home. You are in your own home. You are in the hallway, so you might as well go for a walk up the drive."

He said, "Oh yes, that's where I was going."

He does not like to admit he forgets these things. He will still try to cover his memory loss up. Two minutes later he was still stood in the hallway and wondering where he was.

Sometimes he gets so confused. He can never find a walking stick even though he has about six of them. I find them in the most stupid of places, including under the settee and on the drive. I even found one enclosed in the shower curtain and one wrapped in a bath towel. The same goes for his hat and glasses – I have found them in the fridge. It seems to me like he hides them away – they are his property. The only trouble with that is that sometimes he can't find them again until weeks later.

I can never do my daily chores at ease, as I have to be watching him all the time, especially when he is moving around, because he loses his balance and is liable to fall down. He cannot use a frame to walk with because of his weak left arm and foot – there is no strength in them – so it has to be a walking stick. Thank goodness his right arm is very strong.

When he goes for his walk up the drive I will leave him to it, but I watch him out of the window because if he goes out of the gate he loses his way. One day he only walked past two bungalows and I could see he was lost.

I went after him and asked him, "Where are you going?"

He said, "I am lost. I cannot find my home. Can you help me find my wife?"

I smiled at him and pointed at myself. I said, "Look, I am your wife. Come on, I will take you back to your home."

I got hold of his bad arm and took him back in and gave him a cup of tea to settle him.

One day when we were having a walk in the park I saw an elderly gentleman fall down. I helped him to his feet and sat him on the park bench. He had cut his head (not badly). I could see he was dazed and confused. I asked him where he lived and his name because I knew he had banged his head when he fell. He did not know his name, and he did not know where he lived and couldn't tell me where he was going. I could see he was the same as my husband – a dementia sufferer. I rang for an ambulance and they took care of him. I thought to myself, 'If my husband ever manages to get away from me I hope whoever finds him takes him somewhere he is safe.'

My two daughters visit me sometimes on a weekend. We have a chat and a cup of tea and a good laugh. One day they told me in no uncertain terms, "Goodness, you're getting fat."

I agreed. "Yes, I have put a stone in weight on."

Although I always watch what I give Francis to eat I had let myself go. I was comfort eating because I was feeling sorry for myself and I could not do things I used to. I had to spend all of my time looking after Francis. Because of his sickness and ailments, he needed my constant attention day and night.

Before his sickness I used to cycle ten miles every day and go swimming twice a week. I had freedom to come and go as

I pleased. Now I feel I am in prison and my life is spoken for. I feel useless and fat.

They told me that if I didn't look after myself and stay healthy the pair of us would be finished. Who would look after him then? They brought me to my senses. I resolved to find a couple of hours a week of respite for him and me, so he could communicate with others like him and I could do a bit of keep fit and, with a bit of luck lose the stone in weight I had gained and recharge my strength.

STRENGTH TO CARRY YOU THROUGH

When I see you struggling along,
When all you touch turns out so wrong,
Pity and love I feel for you,
Knowing what you need to do,
Giving you strength to carry you through.

You are a lovely, placid man,
Always trying the best you can,
Always proud and kind, that's you,
Happy in everything you do,
Giving you strength to carry you through.

As you go along your way,
Spreading joy from day to day,
Passing everyone with a smile,
Making them cheerful for a while,
Giving you strength to carry you through.

Thoughtful you have always been,
Attempting things you are so keen.
You say good morning and good day
To anyone who goes your way,
Giving you strength to carry you through.

Never complaining no matter what,
So contented with your lot.
What comes your way you always try,
Never stopping to wonder why,
Giving you strength to carry you through.

When I see you struggling along,
When all you touch turns out so wrong,
Pity and love I feel for you,
Knowing what you need to do,
Giving you strength to carry you through.

Francis's memory gets worse as the weeks go by. It is so distressing for me to see. He is forgetting me and our family and leaving us behind for longer periods at a time. It is like his mind is dying slowly.

The hardest thing for me is knowing he cannot get any better in his mind. This is so hard to accept, but I know for his sake and mine I have to. I watched him going through it day after day, night after night. To see this happening to a loved one, knowing nobody can help him, is heartbreaking. I have cried myself to sleep on many a night. A carer needs a good weep – it washes the stress away. Everything seems to wash out of your system, giving you strength to carry on. It is like a new day has begun. You can face anything – bring it on!

I have *The Telegraph* delivered for him every day because he reads it after a fashion. When he has finished reading it he will say I can have a read, but the state I get it in there is not much chance of that! I cannot put it back together again. It will be all screwed up and flung around the floor. I always ask him to let me read it first, but he never does.

Sometimes I look at what he has spent half an hour reading and I ask him to tell me what it was about. He reads me a report, but it has nothing to do with what he has just read.

He sometimes sits reading a book for hours at a time. He

has been reading the same book for at least two years now and he is still on page two!

I ask him, "Is that a good book?"

He will say, "Oh yes, it is excellent!"

I say, "Oh, good. What is it about, then?"

He will make a story up, and the story he makes up is always a war story, but the book is nothing to do with the war. I don't say anything to him about that because I know he has to believe in himself and while he is sat reading it gives him something to occupy himself with.

Sometimes I let him wash the pots and make himself a cup of tea. This way he thinks he's being a help to me. He likes to think he is useful and still a man, even though I have to wash them again later without him seeing me because I don't want him to feel bad about himself because he cannot manage to do it right.

Like me he has no freedom to come and go like he used to, so he must also feel the same as me. That's why he gets so upset and frustrated at times.

It is a good thing that he cannot remember most things, because then nothing plays on his mind like it does on mine. I do notice that sometimes he has been crying – I can tell by his eyes.

We had a cat. She was a lovely, happy cat, friendly with both of us, especially with him. She behaved like a dog – she followed him everywhere. When he went for his walk she walked alongside him; when he stopped walking so did she. She would sit down looking at him, waiting for him to start walking again, then off they would go again. If he stopped to talk to the neighbour over the fence she sat there waiting patiently for him. When they came back in the house and he sat on his chair she would jump up on to his knee at every chance she got. She was always by his side.

I had to give her away to a good family – I had no choice. I cried for days after she had gone because she was part of our family. I hated having to give her up, but it was for her own good. It was so she would not get hurt because if he was in the bathroom she would sit and sleep on his chair and when he went to sit down on it he would not lower himself down; he would just drop straight down with all of his weight straight on to the poor cat, never stopping to look if she was on there first. Many a time I had to take her to the vet to make sure he had not broken any of her bones. I was always telling him to watch out for her, but with his dementia he never did and I could not watch his every movement. He did it so many times – he could never remember to look out for her on his chair. He would always say sorry, and I know he was. It hurt him to think he might have hurt her.

He would always say, "I cannot remember. I am sorry."

So for her own health she had to go, because I know he would have never forgiven himself if he had hurt her. He loved cats, and he had always had one. He never mentioned her after she was gone. We do have a few other cats that come into our garden, and he always strokes them and will smile at them through the window.

He will say to me when one appears, "Look, the black cat has come in our area." And then he will go outside and stroke it.

I don't know about him being confused and not being able to work things out sometimes – he confuses me! One day I will ask him to write down his signature; he will and it will be perfect. Then another day it will be a load of scribble that nobody would be able to understand or make out. He will write something down, and he can read it, but when I look at what he has written I cannot read it because it is a line of scribbly words, just like a child who is learning to write. And that's what I think of when he's trying to dress himself or mend something: he is trying to do things that he did when he was a child, having to learn all over again.

I take him for a haircut every couple of months. He always feels happy and confident in himself after he has been there because I make sure he pays for it himself on his good days. They are good hairdressers because they are dementia-friendly. They make sure he does not fall, and they make him feel good, telling him he looks rather young with his new haircut and I must watch him because all the young women might run off with him.

I always say, "They can have him, but not his pension."

I could not believe my luck – we had no appointments written down for the next two weeks – freedom for both of us. No hospitals, no clinics, no doctors, no nurses! We only live once, so I decided we were going to live dangerously. We would drive up to Scotland, and we would be going the scenic way, stopping whenever we felt like it along the way. I booked a B & B in Dornoch, Scotland, for seven days.

He enjoyed the ride up. I stopped every two hours for breaks. The scenery was fantastic and he never complained of one ailment. He told me he was loving his holiday. We booked in and spent a couple of days looking around Dornoch. We stood watching a Scottish band in all their kilts and he pointed out the colourful tartan, which was that of the Black Watch. Taking advantage of his fitness, because his health was fine, I drove on to a ferry which took us to the Isle of Oban, which we drove around. Sheep just wandered across our path. We stopped to look at the mountains and waterfalls, then we had dinner in a hotel and caught the ferry back to our B & B.

We stayed until our week was up, then started for home. We had not been driving for long when a pickup truck loaded with pallets of cans of beer lost half its load right in front of us. The pallets just slid off the truck. Luckily for us they landed on the grass verge – the wind had taken them to the side of us. Talk about living dangerously! I think our guardian angel looked after us that day. No one was hurt, and the truck kept going and so did we, but the traffic behind us did not. They stopped and filled their cars up with the cans of beer. They must have thought it was Christmas – and well, come to think of it, it was for them. It had taken me a while to realise what had happened in front of me and to get over the shock of it. If I had thought of it sooner I would have been right alongside them filling my car up too. When their family asked them how they came to have a car full of cans of beer and they told them they fell off a lorry, they would have laughed at them, not believing it could be true. My family tell me I am slow to catch a cold.

My daughter said, "Was it worth taking him when he does not even remember where he has been or what he has done? He will say he has had an excellent time, but can never say why and he does not have any memories of it to think about."

I told her, "It did him a world of good. He was happy and relaxed, and he never complained once. He had no ailments between going and coming back. He looks well and feels good and he had plenty of fresh air and enjoyed it at the time. The same goes for me. So yes, it was well worth going – it was something different for us."

While the sun lasts I have found a good way of relaxing for ten minutes. One day I went into the conservatory to dust, and when I had finished I rested there for ten minutes. The heat hit me, and I was sat there sweating. I thought, 'This is good. This is like going to the sauna that I used to go to and I don't even have to go out of my own door. I don't have to leave him.' I could not have asked for a better way to spend ten minutes of 'me time'. When I went back into the living room to check on Francis, he was sat quite contentedly reading a book. I told him that I would be having a sauna in our conservatory when the sun was out and he would be banned from there because it would be my ten minutes of 'me time'.

He said, "Oh, good – you can trust me. I will watch television or read my paper."

I knew I could not trust him, but I would still have my sauna. I would just make sure he was settled and the door was locked before I did.

He had four weeks of good days – I could not believe my luck!

– then it was back to bad days and maybe weeks of them.

I had just given him a shower, put his nightclothes on and settled him down watching the television while I cooked the tea. I had just about finished it when I saw water coming towards me, heading for my feet. I ran into the bathroom, where he was stood holding the door of the bath open and water was pouring out of it. His dressing gown and slippers were off – they were on the floor, floating around with the bath mat. He told me he had closed the door of the bath, filled it up with water to have a bath, then opened the door to get in it (which he had forgotten to do). I turned off the taps and pulled out the plug to let the water out – it was just about gone anyway, into the hallway and kitchen.

I was angry. I had to count to ten. I told him, "I have only just given you a shower. You are never to have a shower or bath ever again without me being with you!"

He knew he had done something wrong. He said, "Oh! I'm sorry – I did not know I had already had a shower."

I dressed him once again, sat him back in the living room and gave him his tea. I thought, 'While he is eating I can get everything dried up.'

But he kept coming into the hallway, standing in the water, saying sorry. He did that a couple of times while I was trying to get it done. I had to shout at him to get him to sit down so he did not slip. I told him that I did not want to have to take him to hospital if he slipped. It worked – he sat down reading.

Later we both had a cold tea. I told him I was sorry for shouting, but I did not want him falling. He said he was sorry (he had done this twice in a week).

I said, "It is not you, it is your sickness."

He said, "Oh, I know I don't remember things. I always forget. I'm sorry."

I felt guilty for shouting. I was not shouting out loud – I was talking between gritted teeth before I counted to ten.

Now and again we visit one of my friends. She had a stroke,

but it did not leave her with brain damage. It left her with a weak heart and paralysed left arm and leg, but she is doing quite well. She is able to get around on her mobility scooter, which is a good thing because she lives on her own.

If we don't have much to do and are out and about in the area where she lives we call in for a chat and a cup of tea to see how she is getting on.

Francis is not too keen on visiting her because she takes the mickey out of him and she is not happy until she makes him blush.

She starts on him the minute we get inside her door. She will say to him, "I need some company – just a companion. You will do because you have a nice smile." We have a chat and a drink, and if she has not managed to make him blush or feel uneasy she will have another go at him. She will say, "Come and live with me. We can go to the park, and you can ride on my scooter. Don't worry about what she will say – she is my friend, and friends should share. Don't let her moan at you. If she does I will deal with her. Her mother always said she was a moaning Minnie. If she throws you out come to me. I will take you in, but don't forget to bring your tranquillity bath with you. Then we can both have a spa together."

That does it for sure. He will go bright red and start to choke. He tries to get out of there as fast as he can. I have to stop him from falling over. She will double up with laughing and grab his hand to help him out.

I will say to her as we are leaving, "Leave him alone, you rotter! He is mine – you cannot have him."

She will say, "Let me have him for one week and you can have him for one week. He will be safe with me. He will be looked after like a king. It will give you a break. I won't moan at him."

He drags his arm away from her, stumbling and falling about, getting into the car as fast as he can to get away from her. Then he locks the door (even with his memory he does not forget to do that!).

She shouts after him as we leave, "I like a man that blushes."

I often wonder if she is kidding.

He sees the nurse every week for his INR jab to check his blood count to see how thick or thin his blood is. He had blood clots on his lungs, so he has to take warfarin. You would think he would be used to it by now, but every time she touches his finger to click it on he shouts and jumps a foot in the air, making me and the nurse jump also. It does not make any difference if she tells him it's coming or not, the minute she puts it on his finger that's it – he jumps. Then she jumps and drops the finger needle every time. Once his blood count returns to a safe level it won't have to be monitored every week; we will have a couple of weeks' rest. When that happens, like me the nurse will be glad of a short break. Every time we see her he behaves like a child.

I tell him, "Don't watch what she is doing." And I say, "Goodness me, it is only a little prick." But he still jumps – it is the thought of it. It is the same when we have our flu jabs. He makes me have mine first, making out he is being a gentleman, but it is because he does not like needles and, like most men, he has to show how brave he is.

We have to be careful what we say in front of him because he cannot always work out what people are saying.

One day when one of my daughters came to visit us she said, "I have just passed an accident. Someone with a car the same colour and make as yours has just crashed into a tree."

Francis looked at me and started shouting and pointing at me in an aggressive manner while walking backwards and forwards. Then he stopped near me and stared at me, waving his good arm up and down. He shouted at me, "What have you done with the car? Why has the car hit a tree? Why have you crashed the car?"

We were both trying our best to calm him down, telling him, "Look, I am here – I have not been in the car today. I have been with you. It was somebody else who has done that."

But he would not calm down, no matter what we said. We

took him outside and showed him the car on the drive, and that calmed him for a while, but all night he was insisting I had crashed the car and the car had hit a tree. It tickled me, but we all agreed to try not to mention things like accidents in front of Francis. But it is hard to remember when we are talking together.

As time goes by Francis gets harder for me to handle. I will help him wash, dress and shave, give him his breakfast, then settle him down with a book or in front of the television so I can shower and get dressed myself, but on occasions he won't let me.

He will follow me around, rapping his walking stick on the ground impatiently, repeating over and over again, "Come on, we have to go out. We have to go now."

So I have to stop whatever I am doing to try and settle him again, constantly telling him we don't have to go out. In the end I have to tell him off in a stern voice, just like telling off a child who has done wrong. Then I finish getting myself ready. When I go to check on him he will have thrown most of his clothes around the house like a spoilt child would. So I tell him off like one, and I make him pick everything back up and put them back where he got them from. He knows he should not have done that. He picks them up and puts them back (in a fashion) and he will tell me he is sorry.

On a very bad day (which he has plenty of) he does not want to do anything. I know it is because he is not feeling too good – these are the days when he loses his balance and needs extra help. He will wobble around and drop down with all his weight on anything or anyone when he sits down. He won't even attempt to help himself. When I am lifting him up and down, he will be a dead weight, hanging on to anything. That's when I use his indoor wheelchair and make him grab hold of it to walk him around to keep him going. I still tell him to wash himself, which he does in the sink while sat in his chair – at least he *tries* to wash. After a couple of these bad days he will do his best and he will get back on his feet, attempting most things himself. I always win – I get him moving one way or another.

While he is sat I massage his legs. I force his legs up and down and I tell him to move his arms about. I do this to make sure he does not seize up altogether (he will do this soon enough). As soon as he regains his strength he has his twenty minutes' tranquillity spa bath, which makes him healthy – it circulates his blood around his body.

At this stage of the game it is best I care for him on my own, with my family helping when I need them, because I don't have to stick to certain times; things don't have to be done to order. Having seen to him, it will be dinner time before I know it and I can see to myself any time of the day. When I have appointments I can work around them. If I had someone coming in to help me it just would not work out. Because he has so many clinic and hospital visits we could not stick to their times and they would be in my way. So until I find it too much to handle I'm quite happy to do it my way. I might not get everything done on time, but I do get it done.

Francis is my first priority – everything else is not so important, even me. I do know there is so much help out there for patients and carers whenever I feel the need for it. Doctors and nurses do their very best to help patients stay in their own homes. They all deserve gold medals for what they do and achieve. But up to now Francis is staying with me.

Sometimes I tell myself I deserve a medal for what I have to do and go through, because every day and night he tortures my brain. It feels like he brainwashes me. He always asks me the same things over and over again. Even when I give him the answer, that won't stop him. I write down the answer to whatever he is asking and when he repeatedly wants an answer I pass him the reply on the paper. He will read it, and on the bottom of the reply I write in large writing, 'I have told you this ten times and I am not telling you again. I am not a parrot.'

Then he looks at me and says his favourite saying, "Oh, I am sorry. But you should have told me this in the first place, because it is the first time I have heard of it."

Then I am forever giving him the paper it is written on or telling him to read it again, but even that does not stop him.

Another way is to make him think of something else, to make him forget what's on his mind. Mostly I take him out or tell him to have his walk up the drive. Sometimes I feel guilty again with myself – I think it is ironic that here I am trying to make him forget!

It must have been two o'clock in the middle of the night, and I realised he was not in bed. I could not hear any noise or movement, so went to look for him. I found him in the living room. I had to turn on the light because it was pitch-black. He was sat in his chair. He had his glasses on and was reading the paper.

I asked him, "What are you doing sat in the dark?"

He said, "I am reading the paper."

I said, "You cannot read without the light on – it's dark in here."

He jumped up and threw his glasses on to the chair, saying, "Oh, yes I can. I don't even need glasses. I always read in the dark."

I said, "Oh, you are clever. Have you got X-ray eyes or is it because you eat carrots? I will leave the light on so you can see what you are reading."

He started waving his arms around, getting quite agitated, saying, "I can read it – I don't need the light."

I had to calm him down. I said, "It's OK. I wish I had perfect eyes like you – you are so lucky. But do you know what time it is? We have to go to sleep because we have appointments tomorrow."

He went to bed and slept.

We always watch *Coronation Street* and most of the other soaps – we have for years.

We sat watching one night when he said to me, "I enjoyed that film. I want to see it again if possible because it is the first time I have seen that famous actor for two years."

I told him, "You are in luck, then, because it is on again tomorrow so we can watch it again."

Another time, when we were watching a football match he said to me, "How are we going to get home? Where is the car? How did we get to this match? I don't know this street. I don't know how to get home." He was looking anxious and frightened.

I explained to him, "We are at home – we are watching the match on television."

He got quite angry. "I am watching it with all these people. Where is the car? I want to go home."

I took his hand. "Come with me. I will show you that you are in your own home."

I showed him the hallway, the kitchen and his bedroom.

He said, "Oh, good."

So we sat down again to watch the match.

Then he said, "Oh, it is good that they are playing in my area, but how will we get home?"

I could not make him understand that we were not at the match, so I turned the television off and he sat reading a book. He did not mention it again.

He enjoyed his day out in the park one day because we met three of our great-grandchildren there. They were playing on the swings.

He recognised them immediately, waving and saying to me, "Look, some of ours."

I pushed him near so he could sit and watch them. I'm not surprised he recognised them because we have photographs of them all around the living room and I tell him who they are nearly every day. They waved and shouted at him to watch them sliding down the slide. They ran up to him and told him to watch how they could climb up the climbing wall, telling him they could reach the top and that they were only five years old – twins. They made sure he was watching by waving to him. He clapped and cheered them on. Their older brother did football tricks and threw the ball to him to catch. He could not manage to catch it – his reactions were not quick enough – but he tried. He was so proud and happy to have spent some time with them.

Well, one day I left him to his reading. He had had a good bath, eaten his breakfast and had his medication. I locked the door. Now it was my turn – I was having my sauna in my conservatory and it was great. I felt quite peaceful and relaxed. It was my ten minutes of 'me time', although I was listening for movement from him in case he got up to something he should not be doing – over the last six years he had done plenty of that. All was still, and I could feel the tension going out of me.

After my ten minutes was up I checked him. He was snoring away with his reading book in his hands, so I even managed to have a shower in peace without having to run about after him.

Here we go again. Francis had a fungal infection on his toenails, and the doctor gave me some cream to put on them, but that is more easily said than done. I would go as far as to say it is almost impossible, because Francis won't let me get anywhere near his feet. He is so ticklish that every time I try he pulls his feet away and breaks out in hysterics. He could not put the cream on himself because he was going through his bad days and he could not bend his knees. At last I managed it with great difficulty. I went through the same thing for a full week. I have never laughed so much in my life, and neither has he. Eventually the infection cleared up. But what is it I always say? As fast as one ailment is gone another takes its place.

This time it was toes again – chilblains – so I had another week of trying to get cream in between his toes. So every morning for two weeks we were both hysterical with laughter.

Looking after him all these years, with his sickness and my age, does nothing to keep wrinkles at bay. It takes its toll because I have no time to myself to look after my skin or health, and health is something you should never neglect. We should always find time for ourselves.

When I used to bump into friends while out and about they would say to me, "You never change – you always look twenty years younger than you are and healthy and happy." But ever since I began looking after Francis, spending all my time on him, it had been a lot different. They didn't say it any more, and by the look on their faces I got the feeling they felt sorry for me. But they still told him how young and healthy he looked after all he had been through. When I looked in the mirror I could understand why, because I saw a tired, drained face with more lines on it than a writing pad. What else should I expect? I should be taking it easy at my age! But then I told myself I had good health compared to Francis, so why should I not look good like I used to? So I changed, I had a nice hairdo and looked after my skin, putting plenty of cream on. I felt better myself because I was also spending time on me. I felt happy with myself and did not feel resentful towards Francis, which I used to. In my mind I was blaming it on him, but it was not his fault I was letting myself go; it was me. He had always tried his best, so now I was trying my best.

After a few weeks of looking after myself it worked. When I bumped into old friends they would say, "You look young – tell me your secret. How do you do it?"

I would say, "Oh, it does not take much doing – just be happy with yourself and your life. Spare yourself a little time and keep putting on your cream."

As well as looking after myself I also take two hours a day to do a bit of writing. I have been writing poems mostly. It gives me something else to think about, to occupy my mind. I have to have something to take my mind off caring, to keep me sane, because dementia sufferers play with your mind if you let them. You can doubt your own sanity, especially when you are with them all the time. Listening to them repeating themselves, asking you over and over the same question! You answer them, but they never take it in. You are constantly trying other ways to pacify them. You cannot talk to loved ones about what you go through because they have their own families to care for. It is my burden to carry; they will have enough of their own throughout their life.

There is plenty of help out there for carers – you just have to find it. A problem shared is half the load. Plus, in my experience, it is helpful to talk with someone who knows all about vascular dementia. It makes me feel I am not on my own, because sometimes that is how I feel. Also, when I have done some little thing for Francis and he looks up at me and says thank you, then I know I am not alone.

YOUR ONLY ONE TRUE LOVE

One day will come your one true love
Sent to you from heaven above,
The only one who is meant to be,
Coming the once to you and me.
You will know when your love appears.
Never let it disappear –
Your one true love.

A love to last for evermore,
A love that you would die for,
Feeling contented, feeling the joy,
Feeling happiness, feeling lots more,
Your soulmate, your friend for life,
Your husband or your wife –
Your only one true love.

Someone that you hold dear,
Someone to keep near,
One who thinks the world of you,
One who always will be true.
Don't ever send your love away,
Regret it you will day by day –
Your only one true love.

Lose your love, it won't come again.
Lose your love, you will feel the pain.
You will be downhearted, lost and alone;
You will be broken, a lost lonely soul.
A needing, a caring that no one would see,
A longing, a yearning for what used to be –
Your only one true love.

One day will come your one true love
Sent to you from heaven above,
The only one who is meant to be,
Coming the once to you and me.
You will know when your love appears.
Never let it disappear –
Your only one true love.

I was congratulating Francis. Over the last four weeks he had been so good – he was no trouble to me at all. I had plenty of sleep and rest as he had only been up a couple of times throughout the nights. It was like heaven. I would have been beginning to look on him as being back to his normal self if it had not been for the way he dragged himself around. I thought the dementia had gone, had left him. He was even doing his walks up the drive four times a day without me having to tell him to, even dressing himself and fastening buttons up in the right holes. No problems, no aches and pains. But in the back of my mind I told myself not to count chickens before they hatch, and I was proven right.

The bombshell hit one night after we had gone to bed. I awoke at twelve and he was not in bed. I found him lying on the floor – he had fallen. I asked him what had happened. He was looking dazed and was trying to tell me, but all that was coming from him was a load of rubbish. I could not understand what he was trying to tell me. I checked him over. He was not bleeding. I put a pillow under his head and called the ambulance.

They got him sat up in the chair to examine him, and by then he had come round a lot. He told them in a slurred voice that he had fallen down. He said he was not hurt, but he must go now because he was going to the army barracks to see his wife. I was there in the bedroom with him, plus it had been over forty years since he was in the army.

The paramedics could get no sense out of him. Although they could see he didn't appear to have hurt himself, they couldn't be sure he hadn't had a mini stroke as he had had two strokes before and a bleed on his eye from a previous fall, so they took him to hospital for a check-up.

He was checked over and thankfully I could take him back home, but not before he had two more ailments to add to his list: a water infection and a bad cold. This meant more appointments to see the nurse, and to add insult to injury he gave me his cold.

That was the start of him going back in time again to when he was in the army, which was to last for at least two months. He was always wanting to go to the barracks and wanting his passport. I had to keep reminding him he did not have to go anywhere because he was retired from the army and was now a pensioner.

He would just laugh at me. "Never! I never am!"

Well, I could not bring him back to reality, so while he was thinking he was there I thought I would find out a bit about his army days, because I was not with him then. I knew he had done twenty years' army service from the age of seventeen in the Royal Engineers. He told me he was building bridges and was on Christmas Island and had to watch the atomic bomb go off with other young soldiers. He would teach soldiers to shoot, and he became a sergeant. He also went to Thailand and Singapore and was in Londonderry, Ireland, and Germany. After he left the army he became a prison officer down south, and he told me he often had to escort many famous murderers to court, but he did not see anything spectacular about working in the prisons and was always happy to be going home after his shifts. I could not believe how much he remembered, seeing as he had dementia – it must have been because he was reliving his life again.

When we go out for the day, shopping, I always make sure he has money in his wallet so he can buy himself something. It helps him to feel independent and happy. I like him to buy himself a book to read, but he always ends up buying socks and I can never stop him. I tell him he has two drawers full of them. I end up taking bags full of them to the charity shops, and if he catches me giving them away he gets very angry and annoyed and will say, "They are mine. I have not got any socks left."

So I have to give them away when he cannot see me.

Before bed he will often say, "What are we doing tomorrow?"

I don't tell him as a rule because it stays in his mind all night, but sometimes I slip up and tell him. One night I said we had to go out, but not early – not until he has had his dinner. I realised I had slipped up by telling him.

He shook me awake at two in the morning. He was all ready to go, saying, "Come on, it is time to go." He had his trousers on over his nightclothes, and he had his shoes on without his socks. He did have his hat on and had hold of his stick, but he had no coat, only his pyjama top. He was shouting, "Come on, we have to go."

I had to settle him down, saying, "Yes, we have to go, but not just yet. It is too early. We have to have some sleep first, then we can go, so get back into bed."

He took his shoes and trousers off, then put his stick down, got back into bed and went to sleep with his hat still on his head.

In the morning I got up and left him sleeping until I had made the breakfast. When I went into the living room I stood there in shock. He must have been up half the night trying to dress himself. There were nearly all the clothes from out of his wardrobe spread around on the floor and chairs and a couple of pairs of his shoes. It was no wonder he was fast asleep when I woke up.

It must have taken me an hour to put everything back in its place – that was all I needed to start my day!

I woke him up after making his breakfast and he had the

cheek to tell me he was tired.

I told him, "Yes, and so am I after clearing all your clothes away after you pulled out the drawers again."

His reply was "What, me? I have been asleep, and I have had a good night's sleep."

Whatever!

I have found his clothes in the kitchen cupboards before. When I ask him why he puts his clothes in the kitchen with the pots, he will say he has been tidying up the house for me. What can I say after that?

Every morning we get the same carry-on. He has an electric razor because it is easier for him to shave himself. With an ordinary one he would nick himself, and with him being on warfarin it would be hard to stop him bleeding. Before he starts to shave himself he will stand there looking at me with his shaver in his hand, moving it up and down, saying, "This is broken – it will not go."

I go over and switch it on for him.

He will smile. "Oh, it is OK – I have mended it."

I say, "Good for you. I'm glad you got it going." And I praise him. I think he does it so I will thank him for it.

We were relaxing watching television one day when he got up, put his hat on, picked up his walking stick and said, "Where are the car keys? I will take you for a drive."

I have to explain to him, "You cannot have the car keys – you have no car. Your licence was stopped because you have dementia and cannot remember how to drive. You have not driven for six years."

That was the first time in all those years that he had wanted to drive.

He said to me, "I want my licence and car keys."

I told him, "Don't ever think of driving that car on the drive because it is not ours – I just let my friend park there."

He kept insisting I give him the car keys so he could drive off. I explained how sick he was and told him how long he was in hospital and how sick he still is.

He said, "Oh no, I never was. I am as fit as any man. I can drive."

He gets quite angry with me, so I tell him it's bath time and I help him to bathe to take his mind off it, hoping he forgets about wanting to drive.

One month he went back to the days when he worked as a prison officer. He kept asking me, "When am I going back to work?"

I asked him, "What work are you wanting to go to?"

"To the prison service. I must go to the station to check train times."

And so for a vast number of times I tried telling him, "You don't work any more – you have not worked for years. You are a pensioner, same as me."

But no matter what I say to him he cannot retain it. I waste my time. I knew this, but I tried because I knew he was in a phase of wanting to wander off and he would try until he went on to something else.

I know each different phase he goes through will last at least a month. Sometimes whatever I do or say will not pacify him at all. I feel I am beaten. He will sit there getting quite mad, rapping his cane on the floor, looking confused, trying to work things out, repeating himself over and over again. "I must go on the train. I have to go to work."

When all else fails I take him out for the day, and while we are out he forgets about it until he comes back home. Then it starts again.

He had put his own channel on the television and was sat there enjoying it, smiling and saying to me, "This is a great film. That actor is a great fellow. I have seen him before in this film, but I cannot remember his name."

I smiled at him. He had the selling channel on – they sell goods all day long. The man he was on about was selling brushes.

209

I said, "Yes, that man is a good top actor. Yes, you have seen this film before – I watched it yesterday with you. It is a repeat."

He said, "Oh, did we? I don't remember."

I turned the channel over to a war film. He was happy with that. I was not going to sit there all night watching them advertising goods. That's what he turns on every time I let him choose what he wants to watch. I don't like to turn it over after I have told him he can pick the channel, but once I tell him we have both seen the film he usually does not like to admit to me that he does not remember. I sometimes feel guilty about pulling the wool over his eyes, but I do it in a nice way – a way that is better for the pair of us.

Some days he gets so frustrated and agitated because he cannot do things he used to when he was fit. On those days I find him something to occupy his mind, so he does not have time to sit around feeling sorry for himself.

If his balance is not too bad I will spend time in the garden with him. He will pull a few weeds up, and it makes him feel like he's doing something useful.

I praise him by telling him, "You made a good job of that. It looks much better now." And he is happy.

When he has done his bit of gardening he will relax in the living room and read a book or his paper, then after tea I let him help do the washing-up, even though I do it again later on. For him he has had a hard day's work and he falls asleep in his chair – at least it has stopped him feeling frustrated and upset with himself. It makes him feel helpful instead of feeling useless.

Some days if I miss the paper woman I push him in his wheelchair to the paper shop. It is a nice walk there, but coming back it is a steep hill. He enjoys the scenery, but for me, when we get home – well, I am shattered.

When I had our walk-in bath fitted I thought it the best thing we had ever done. After he has had a bath he looks so fit and healthy, and the same goes for me. Sometimes I wonder if it is the best thing I did, because every time he gets out of the bath, instead of grabbing the handrail to pull his fourteen stone up, he will grab the taps, which are only six inches below.

I tell him time and time again, "Grab the handrail, not the taps."

He will say in an aggressive manner, "I always do." Even though I have just seen him do it in front of me.

I can see it won't be long before he pulls the taps off, but I have resigned myself now to it, knowing they will be pulled off sooner or later. It's not his fault. I tell myself taps can be replaced, but he cannot. And it does make us both feel good – so yes, it was worth it.

I had to drag him out of bed one morning as he was struggling to even sit up. When I asked him what was wrong with him and was he hurting anywhere he said he had a pain in his stomach and a pain in his back near his waist.

I thought, 'This is something new. It's the first time he has had stomach ache and back pain. It is usually his legs when he cannot get out of bed. Oh well, there is a first time for everything.'

Anyway, I got him on his feet and he carried on with his walk up the drive. I told him we would see if it makes his stomach ache go away. He took both of his walking sticks, even though one of them does not touch the ground. He carries it two feet from the floor because he has no strength in his left arm to lean on it, but he says it helps him with his balance. So who am I to deny this – whatever helps him out!

All day I kept a close eye on him, worrying myself sick in case he was really sick again. I know he has chronic kidney disease, and I was a bit frantic with watching him, hoping he was all right. All day he continued going outside, but he only stood on the doorstep, closing the door behind him. I was suspicious, so the next time he did it I stood listening on the other side of the door. I soon found out what he was up to –

what was causing him his pain. I heard him: he was blowing off wind! So that was his secret – the reason he was in and out of the door.

I thought to myself, 'You might have lost your memory, but you can remember to hide things from me.'

After he had run in and out of the door like the clappers, remembering to close the door after him, I challenged him. I said, "No wonder you have stomach ache! No wonder you keep legging it in and out of the door, gasping for fresh air! It is because you are full of wind. Well, you are not sleeping in this house tonight if you don't get rid of that, because if I breathe that lot in it will see me off and I must think about my own health for once!"

We were both laughing about it.

After he went outside a few more times he said, "It is all right now – you can breathe in peace. You won't die. All the wind has gone and my belly is free of pain. It has gone."

I thought, 'Yes, I have a bigger pain, and that's you!'

One day he sat there sneezing, so I told him, "Go get yourself a handkerchief from out of your dresser drawer." Later he came back and I asked him, "Did you find the handkerchiefs all right?"

He said, "Of course I did. I'm not stupid, and I know where my handkerchiefs are, don't I?"

Later on he sneezed again and pulled a handkerchief out and blew his nose on it and put it back in his pocket. I never said a word to him – I don't want to be on his back all the time, telling him he gets things wrong – but the handkerchief that he got was a pair of his underpants.

I thought to myself, 'At least they are clean ones.'

One day he will shock me and get it right for a change. At least he always tries hard, but it takes a lot of understanding and patience from me because he needs so much of my help.

Sometimes I feel like I have not got a husband as in his mind he is rarely here with me. I live with sickness and dementia –

his. I am never free from it, day after day, night after night. I cannot even have a conversation with him because he does not know what I'm talking about. He cannot communicate with me. When I say something to him I think he has understood what I'm saying, but I wait for an answer and he just sits there looking confused. Often he cannot think of what to say. He thinks he is having a conversation with me, but all he ever says is, "It is a nice day today, is it not?" Even if it is in the middle of winter and raining or blowing a gale he says it at least ten times throughout the day. "It is a nice day today, is it not?" I tell myself that although at times I feel like I have not got a husband (and in so many ways I have not) at least he is still with me, if not in mind. I know how alone I would feel if he wasn't here at all, so I settle for that.

His legs are so stiff sometimes that he cannot bend his knees, but that does not stop him from cutting his toenails. He will not let me or anybody else touch his feet because he is so ticklish. He cannot bear it. He puts his leg up on the chair and reaches them that way. The trouble is he cuts them too short, then they fester. Then I have to fight him to put cream on them to heal them, which takes days. Then he will do it again. I tell him time after time to leave them alone, but he won't. The minute my back is turned he will go into the bedroom or bathroom and cut them. He can be crafty when he wants, and he can remember to do that. When he wants to he can hide from me to do it because he knows I will try to stop him. He can hide the nail clippers and find them when he needs them. I just cannot see how he remembers these things. Sometimes I think he is so discreet and crafty.

Sometimes I watch him on his bad days and I feel so sorry for him. I think, 'Will his ailments ever stop? As one gets better another takes its place.'

Over the last six years since his first stroke he has had the book thrown at him. People say these things are sent to try us – well, all I can say is he has been well and truly tried.

213

I always think about what my mother would say to us while we were young: "Bad people will pay the price for their sins at some time in their life." And I think to myself, 'Goodness me, if that is true he must have been a bad one at some time in his life!' But I never believed her anyway, and I have never ever seen or heard him say or do a bad thing in all the sixteen years I have known him. All I see is goodness. He has guts and a strong willpower to get through all the sickness and ailments he has been through, and to fight dementia the way he does takes strength – lots of it.

It was dark in the living room. The curtains were still open and the reflections of our red chandelier in our five small windows made it look as though there were five chandeliers hanging outside. Francis kept looking at them and I could see he was puzzled. He kept going to the window and looking out. He did this about five times, his face showing confusion.

Then he said to me, "Them fancy lights outside are very nice, but you must secure them or they will fall down."

I said to him, "Oh, it is all right. There are no lights outside – it is the reflection of this light in the windows."

He had another look outside and said, "Oh yes, but you must secure them."

I tried again to show him what I meant. I stood alongside him, and I said to him, "Who is that man and woman standing outside the window?"

He smiled and said, "That is me and you."

I said, "Yes, but we are not outside, are we? It is only our reflection in the window because it is dark outside."

I could tell by his face he couldn't understand, and he was looking quite troubled and upset, so I gave in trying to explain. I closed the curtains and turned on the television, but it was still on his mind. A few times in the evening he kept going to the window and looking out of the curtains, trying to convince himself nothing was outside. I just left him to it because I knew whatever I said to him I could not bring him to reality.

I had to take Francis to the hospital again – he had pains in his back and waist and I knew it was not wind this time. After tests, and a couple of days later, I could take him home. This time it was a water infection, which cleared up after two weeks on antibiotics.

While we were at the hospital the surgeon, whom we go to every six months, told me, "You must watch out for him because of his stage-three chronic kidney disease. His eight kidney stones are small at the moment, but until they are the cause of his pain, which is not the case at the moment, we need to wait and see and keep up with his six-monthly hospital appointments."

While he was on his two-week course of antibiotics he took to his bed, so I took advantage of that. I decorated the living room and enjoyed doing it. It took my mind off things, and after I had done it I felt good.

Once he was back on his feet, after one of his spa baths he was back to doing his walks up and down the drive.

I told him, smiling and joking, "Once again you are the walking dead!"

Some nights I lie awake crying because I feel so sorry for him. Watching what he is going through when his mind wanders, I think to myself, 'Oh, the poor devil.' And I feel great sadness. Then I tell myself, 'I have no need to feel sorry for him. He is happy and he has me to look after him besides his children, who spoil him so much.' Then I think of all the other dementia sufferers with this cruel sickness who are living on their own. Thank goodness for all the good and caring people who look out for them: doctors, nurses and others. But when I see what Francis goes through I cannot help grieving for others like him, knowing they go through the same thing and I can do nothing. Then I tell myself, 'Francis is my main concern – I cannot grieve for everybody. He is the one who needs my help. He needs all my time and energy.' Then I feel a great calmness, because I know I am doing my best for him, looking after him the way I do. I know I am doing the right thing. I keep him going; I make him strong. I am his lifeline; I am his friend. But it is not only me who helps – his doctors, his nurses and his surgeons also help to keep him strong, and keep him going.

Sometimes I have to cover things up for him. When we are out with friends and he has been to the toilet, with his left arm being so useless he sometimes comes back with a mark on his trousers. He has not been able to pull them out of the way, and I can see he is embarrassed, trying to cover it with his hand. I pull his jumper over it, or I will say, "Oh, you have splashed water on yourself while washing your hands. Never mind – it is because of your weak hand, you cannot do much with it."

Then we all pass it off and he always looks relieved, but I always think to myself, 'Should I have mentioned it or should I not have drawn attention to it?' I can never know if I am doing the right thing; sometimes I may only think I am.

His nurse always tells him he is spoilt and lucky to have such a good and caring wife; and considering the things I have done for him, and helped him overcome, I think, 'Yes, I could not have helped him any other way.'

He has got to the point where he has illusions. For example, he keeps trying to pick things up off the carpet, but when I look there is nothing there. Then he starts searching around the house, in drawers and under cushions. He walks around the floor, scrutinising, searching, picking things up that are not really there. I get fed up with him searching. I ask him, "What are you looking for? Have you dropped something? Can I help you find it?"

One day he said, "I am looking for an ornament – a small green thing like an animal. I have dropped it and I must find it because it is not mine. I am looking after it for someone. They gave it to me today to mind."

I told him, "But nobody has been here today – only you and me. I have been with you all the time. You have seen it on television."

He said, "I have not. I have to find it – it's on the carpet. I am looking after it for someone."

I settled him down with a cup of tea, thinking he would forget about it, but he went around the house supposedly picking something up off the carpet that was not there. I left him to it, thinking to myself, 'He has been watching the selling channels on TV again!'

I got a date and time to take him for a mental assessment with a specialist about his dementia. This was quite a relief for me – at last someone who knows all about it to discuss things with me!

The specialist assessed him for one hour, asking him to remember things he had told him minutes before, but Francis could not remember most of what he had been told.

The specialist asked him to draw a clock and put a time of two o'clock on the face of it. I looked at what Francis had drawn for him: the clock had the numbers one to thirteen on it written quite shakily, like a three-year-old learning to write for the first time. And when he had written down the time he had only put one hand on it. The big hand was missing.

The specialist asked him if there was anything he had missed out. Francis scrutinised his drawing, checking it over for a while, then said no, he was happy with it.

The specialist told me, "Yes, he has vascular dementia and because it was caused by his strokes there is nothing I can give him to slow it down."

And we were given an appointment for another assessment.

UNTIL WE HAVE TO PART

Through your sickness, your health,
We will find the strength
To carry us through.
No matter what you say or do,
Your love I have within my heart
Until the day we have to part.

Don't worry, I won't leave you.
I will help you on your way.
The two of us will travel your road
Together to share your heavy load.
Doors will close, we might lose our way;
Others will open for a better day.
I look in your eyes and I can see
We will grow stronger, you and me.
You won't carry your burden on your own –
I will be with you, you are not alone.

Tomorrow will be different, you will see –
You can put your trust in me.
As long as I do breathe the air
You will always have me there.
Although I have not known you long
You won't wake up to find me gone.
We will go along our way
Unconcerned by what they say.
We are happy, we are free,
And I hope you always stay by me.

Through your sickness, your health,
We will find the strength
To carry us through.
No matter what you say or do,
Your love I have within my heart
Until the day we have to part.

Francis had had two good weeks and when I looked at the calendar I could not believe our luck – once again we were free for a full four weeks and he had no fresh ailments. Also he was with me in his mind, so to hell with whatever might happen I was taking him on holiday for two full weeks, fully inclusive, to Djerba. We only live once – so off we went.

The airline was very helpful to us. With Francis not able to climb stairs, they took him in their wheelchair through customs and up a lift right to his seat on the plane. It was great for him and me. We got the same treatment when we landed.

We had two weeks of paradise. It did not matter about not being able to go on the beach because we lazed around the swimming pool. Francis could not swim, but I had a swim whenever I wanted one. He kept in the shade, like his nurse told him to, and I kept him well supplied with water, not forgetting his tablets. We even went on excursions to the sand dunes and we had a ride in the desert on a camel cart with a fringe on top. I had a ride on a camel; he did not. Then we both went by Jeep to where *Star Wars* was made. He stayed and sat talking with others who could not climb. He even had a tot of whisky while I looked around the bar that was in the *Star Wars* film.

On the way back to our hotel our bus was stopped and our driver was taken away. We were left wondering what was going on. You can imagine what all of us women were saying to each other. "If we are arrested in a foreign country, we could be locked away for years with nobody knowing where we are. They could do anything to us." We women were really getting panicky and distressed – we might be locked up!

Then another driver came on the bus and explained to us that the driver they took away was being fined because he should not have been driving that bus that day. He was only doing it because he did not want us to not be able to go on our excursion – the driver who was supposed to take us was drunk, so he had stepped in for him – were we relieved about that!

We had to wait for a while, then the driver came back. We all cheered him and made a collection to pay his fine. We carried on back to our hotel, and on the way we stopped to see a desert made of salt. Because of the delay in coming back the tide had come in, so we had to go back to our hotel on a ferry, which was quite scenic. We had a good meal – Francis ate anything he wanted to, and I let him. His diet nurse would have gone grey! Well, we only live once and we were on holiday, and I myself up to now had never stopped eating.

All the full two weeks Francis never complained once and

he never had one ailment. He looked and felt well.

We were driven back to the airport on the bus to come home, and while we were walking to the door of the bus to get off his trousers fell down to his ankles. Although he cannot easily bend his knees, I was dumbfounded because he bent down and pulled them up like greased lightning, even buttoning them back up to make sure they did not drop down again. It was so quick that I was wondering if I was seeing things. I could not have done that as fast.

Everybody was laughing and saying, "Goodness me, mate, you made sure nobody got the chance to see anything."

My oldest daughter met us when we landed, saying, "You both look so fit and healthy."

And we were.

Francis told her he had had an excellent holiday, but he could not remember where he had been or what he had done. But that does not make any difference – the main thing is he enjoyed himself and so did I. And I was happy.

Over the next six months Francis came down quite a lot. His walks up the drive drained his strength. After one he would fall asleep in his chair for nearly an hour at a time, so all those six months he did not do much at all himself.

He had been going back to his army days. Most days he would say to me, "When did we land off the plane?" and "When am I going back off leave?" and "Will I be going back in my uniform?"

It was no good me trying to bring him back to reality because I had tried that so many times previously. After two minutes he cannot retain what I say, so now I leave him to it. I carry on doing whatever I need to do. Telling him the same thing so many times annoys me and stresses me out. I feel guilty sometimes for ignoring what he says, but it is a waste of my time always repeating myself over and over again.

One day we were sat watching television and Francis kept getting up and down, swiping the settee, trying to catch something, then sweeping his good arm in the air.

I thought, 'Goodness me, he has gone crazy! Now what will I do?'

I asked him what was wrong with him.

He said, "It's that shiny thing that's flying around. I cannot catch it. It keeps flying away every time I watch it."

It was the sun reflecting off his watch, around the room.

I laughed and so did he when I said, "You are as bad as the cat – she used to chase after shiny reflections."

I breathed a sigh of relief – at least he had not gone crazy.

He amuses me when I watch him take his tablets – it is the way he takes them.

I tell him, "Always take plenty of water while taking them and put one in your mouth at a time."

He takes a small sip of water, puts the tablet in his mouth, clamps his mouth shut, moves his head from side to side a couple of times, then throws his head forward and gives it a big jerk backwards. Then he pats his belly and opens up his mouth, putting out his tongue to show me the tablet has gone. He gives me a big smile and repeats his actions all over again until all the tablets are gone. I tell him to swallow them one at a time to stop him choking himself, which happens many a time as he finds them hard and dry to swallow.

I am getting used now to the things he says and does. I don't get quite so upset as I used to until he says to me on numerous occasions, "Where is my wife? Where is Iris, my wife?"

It shocks me when he suddenly comes out with that, but then I feel relief because I tell myself that although he has lost me, he still remembers my name. It's a little bit of consolation for me.

Then he says, "Has she gone out and about?"

I point to myself and I ask him, "Who'd you think I am?" feeling quite annoyed.

He will say, "I don't know who you are!" He will look quite frightened and keep asking me where his wife is.

I get sick of repeating myself to him. I feel like a parrot, but he will keep asking me over and over again.

I tell him frantically, "I am Iris, and I am your wife."

But he will still insist, "You are not my wife."

I show him our wedding photographs. I point to myself in a photo and say, "Who is that?"

He will say, "That is Iris."

Then I point to the man and say, "Who is that?"

He will say, "Oh yes, that is me."

Then I tell him, "Yes, that's you and me and we have just been married."

Then a look of relief will come on his face and he will say, "Oh yes, you and me." Five minutes later he will say, "Where is my wife, Iris? Has she gone out and about? When is Iris coming home?"

He has not remembered me for years, so I am flogging a dead horse. There is no way I can get through to him. I look at him with tears in my eyes. I feel so sad for him.

I tell him, "Don't worry. Iris, your wife, won't be long. She will be home soon."

For a while he will say nothing, but his face will be full of torment and fear and he will keep looking out of the window, looking for his wife.

I have lived through a war in fear for my life. I have known hunger and trauma, not knowing if I and my family would die, not knowing if I would ever see my friends again. After what I have seen I should be hard – you would think nothing could hurt me. But I'm not hard. It breaks me up when I see him this way, watching dementia slowly destroying his memory, his mind, taking everything he held dear, and me not being able to comfort him. Nobody is able to help it stop. Sometimes I can soothe him; sometimes nobody can. To him I am no more.

A couple of years ago now we both took out a power of attorney for each other. I am so thankful we did, because now I have to register it with the bank to bring it into force because he cannot deal with his affairs any longer. So now I can get his money out. Because he is so vulnerable, his bank affairs are safer with me. It does not make much difference to him because we have always put our money together. His bank account is used to pay bills; mine is used for food and surplus; and what's left goes into a joint savings account for things we need. We have needed to spend plenty of money since his illnesses, changing lots of things around the house to make it easier for him to get around so he can stay in his own home.

I have to watch his every move. One day he kept on insisting I give him the keys to the car. He knows I hide them from him, along with other keys, for his safety and mine, so he had been searching all through the house all day long. He had asked me to give them to him and was getting quite angry with me when I told him no.

Then he calmed down and said, "You must give them to me. I need to fill the car up with fuel so I can drive to my home." I told him he was already home, and he got angry again, saying, "I want the car keys. I want to drive the car." He was waving his arm around.

I could see I could not calm him, so told him in an angry voice, "You have not got a car and if you ever try to drive my car the police will catch you, and then you will be in trouble because you have no licence." I was in tears, and he could see I was angry.

Then he relented and said, "Oh, I am sorry. I know I am not allowed to drive. I am sorry."

So I told him, "It is only while you are sick. When you get better you will be all right."

He was happy with that.

One day we stayed out shopping nearly all day, visiting family and friends. It was getting late so I thought, 'I will take him for a carvery and I won't have to cook any tea when we get home.'

I filled his plate up with plenty of veg and a couple of chunks of beef. I thought, 'He can leave what he does not want,' because he never eats a large meal anyway. He ate the lot and a pudding, and so did I. We were both fat and full.

On the way home we were both saying, "Oh, my stomach is so full that I wish I had not eaten so much."

We had only been home an hour and were resting when he said, "Are we having tea, then, or are you starving me? It is teatime!"

I nearly choked. I said, "You're joking, surely! We only had that big carvery one hour ago and you were moaning you had eaten too much."

He said, "Oh yes!" and laughed.

I thought, 'He is only having me on.'

Ten minutes later he said, "Are you giving me my tea, then? I am starving hungry."

So to shut him up I made him a sandwich and gave him fruit and a drink. He ate the lot. I felt sick, but I thought to myself, 'At least I have no trouble with him eating.'

After breakfast one morning, still in his pyjamas, he put on a cardigan that had a pocket on each side. He put a small bottle of water in one of the pockets with a comb; in the other one he put two pairs of glasses, his electric razor and a handkerchief.

Then he put his hat on his head and said to me (I was still eating my breakfast), "Come on, then, it is time to go."

I asked, "Where are we going to?"

He said, "We will walk down towards the south coast, then head east, heading for the sea to get the train for home."

I burst out laughing – I could not help it. I felt guilty when I laughed, but I thought it was so funny I could not help laughing and he started laughing with me. I said, in between laughing, "We don't have to go all that way – we are already home." I could see he was confused, so I said, "Come with me – I will prove it." And I took him around, telling him, "That's your bedroom."

He recognised everything and said to me, "I must be loopy, but I wish you would tell me these things. I wish you would tell me I am home."

I tell him, "I have to tell you every day."

He emptied his pockets back out and sat down.

I finished my breakfast, thinking, 'One of these mornings I might get to eat my breakfast while it is hot!'

One of my family said to me after watching him – watching what he says and what he does – "Goodness me, he is a burden – a burden for the rest of his life and yours. I could not do what you do for anything, especially as half the time he does not recognise you or know you are even there."

I agreed with them: "Yes, he is a burden, but it is my burden to bear. I am there for him. At least he is still with me – he is here. I still have a companion, a friend. We are still together even though he does not know it or know me. We go to places together. His grand-bairns love to see him – he is still their great-grandad and grandad. He smiles and knows them when he sees them. They make him feel happy. They like seeing him and I still need him with me. I don't want it any other way. It is hard, I admit, but so what? Sometimes life is hard – not just for me and him. Life is hard for most people. Don't forget, in sickness and in health! And I will carry him for as long as I can, even though he does not know me, and I hope for a few more years yet."

He got up in a right stubborn mood one morning. I knew why – it was because he did not sleep much all night. It was fetch me this, fetch me that. When he did fall asleep he was jumping up all the time, so I never got much sleep either – but then, I hardly ever do.

While helping him wash and dress he was making it so hard for me by keeping his legs stiff, refusing to try and bend his knees and making them very hard for me to lift.

After breakfast I took him out shopping. I was not going to run around after him all day while he was in that mood.

When we got there, as I was getting his wheelchair out of the car he shouted out, "I am not going in that – I can walk. You always make me go in that when I can walk myself."

I told him, "Yes, you can walk, but you can only walk a little way because you are weak with a weak heart valve, which tires you out and makes you breathless."

He was quite angry, shouting at me, "Yes, but I am walking. You always stop me from walking."

I tell him, "You cannot keep your balance – you will fall down."

He was flinging his good arm in the air, getting quite agitated, and I could not get him in the chair.

I said, "OK, then, if that's the way you want it, so be it. Let us see how far you can walk before you fall down and I have to pick the pieces up once again. Let us hope you don't break your other foot with your stubbornness."

It must have taken us half an hour to get to the first aisle in the supermarket. He was out of breath and had gone white, saying, "I cannot walk any further." And he was nearly crying.

I sat him down and went for his chair. I put him in it and took him back to the car, then took him back home. I told him not to get angry with me ever again because it was not my fault he could not walk – it was his sickness. All night he kept saying he was sorry.

We went back to the supermarket the next day and he sat in his wheelchair without saying a word. After doing the shopping I pushed his chair right up to the table in the café and we had dinner. After dinner he kept asking for the toilet. I took him, and we were waiting in a long queue for the disabled one because they were cleaning the others. We must have been waiting ten minutes, and he kept moaning to me that he wanted to go to the toilet. Then all the queue were moaning.

The man in front of me said, "Has anyone tried the door to make sure someone is in there?"

The person in the front of the queue said, "Yes, I did, and it is locked so someone is in there."

Then to prove the point she tried it again and it did not open.

After another five minutes a member of staff came and

knocked on the door. Nobody answered him, so he pushed the door – it opened. It was empty.

He said to the woman, "I thought you said you had tried the door?"

She replied, "I did, but I pulled it instead of pushing it!"

The man in front of me started laughing and said, "Just like a woman, pulling out when she should be pushing in."

When it was his turn I helped him out of his wheelchair and he went into the toilet, I stood waiting outside for him, holding on to his chair.

Then the same bloke who made the joke sat in Francis's wheelchair and said to me, "Is it all right if I take his place? I have always wanted to know what it is like to be pushed around by a woman."

I told him, "I don't think so – this woman is not pushing seconds around, thank you very much. I have enough on my plate to be going on with! Once bitten, twice shy!"

Francis came back and the bloke said to him as he got out of his chair, "I tried to take your place, mate, but she would not let me."

I pushed Francis to the car, and he sat in it reading the paper. I locked him in.

He said to me, "I did not have to wee after all – I did not want one."

After all that moaning and telling me that he could not wait! After waiting in that queue for at least half an hour! I was mad. I could have hit him. Instead I left him there in the car while I did more shopping, taking at least half an hour.

When I got back to the car, which was in the supermarket car park, he had finished reading his paper.

I said, "Have you enjoyed your shopping?"

He said, "Oh yes. Are we going home from our holiday now?"

I said, "What holiday are we on?" (I am used to him thinking he is on holiday when we go out.)

He said, "You know we are on the Isle of Wight. It is very nice here, is it not?" He was smiling.

I said, "Yes, it is great and we are going home right now, today."

I did not want to burst his bubble or try to bring him back to reality because he looked so happy. He looked like he was enjoying himself. I thought, 'Let him think he is on holiday – he is hurting no one. So it is all in his mind – so what!' But I could not help wondering to myself how he could think he was on holiday when we had just been shopping in the supermarket in our own town – something we always do.

One day I left him reading one of his books while I was cooking the tea. When I was finished and took it into the living room for him he was gone. I found him in the bedroom – he had gone to bed with his day clothes on and a pair of boots. He had managed to put his pyjamas on over his boots and all his clothes.

I asked him, "What are you doing in bed?"

He replied, "Because it is bedtime!" And he pulled all the bedding over him, turned over and said, "Night night. I will see you in the morning."

I said, "You are having me on! Do you know it is only four o'clock and I have been in the kitchen cooking your tea? You cannot go to bed at this time of day because you don't sleep very well at night as it is, so get out of that bed right now! And as you managed to put your pyjamas on on top of your clothes and boots by yourself, you can take them back off by yourself. Then come and get your tea!"

I left him to it. I went and had my tea because I was sick of having to eat my meals cold every time because of the things he does and because I was always putting him first.

After a while he came for his tea. He had managed to take his pyjamas back off and still had his boots on. I had a good warm tea; his must have been cold, but he ate it, saying nothing.

My friend – the one who likes to make Francis blush – got him again one day. She made him go red and stumble before we even got into her house. I swear she must keep looking out of her window for us as I believe we make her day.

As we were going up her drive, towards her front door, she rushed out. She grabbed hold of Francis's hand, pulling him towards her door, saying to him, "So, at last you are here to see me, but not before time! What did I tell you to do last time? Well, I told you to come on your own and not to bring her. Now how are we are going to go for a ride on my mobility scooter with her watching? You know I have been waiting and longing for you to come to me. I have been hoping to catch a glimpse of you."

He was trying to shake her hand off him, looking at me pleadingly to help him.

She was telling him, "Oh, no you don't! You are not getting away that easily this time."

I took his hand and said for her to get her own man. He looked quite relieved when I took him home.

This last year he has not been back to me. He has been anywhere and everywhere, but not returned to me. He is back in the army or on his holidays.

When I ask him, "Who are you on holiday with?"

He will say, "I don't know."

One day he kept asking me, "Where has my sister gone? Has she gone back home now?" And he kept looking out of the window, saying, "It is all right, she only lives down the street, round the corner in this area. I saw her cross the road."

I told him, "She lives in Scotland, 300 miles away."

He said, "Oh yes, I know she does, but she just left our house. I was talking to her just today."

I told him, "You are getting a bit confused. She did come to see you not long ago, but she is back home now."

He replied, "Oh yes, I know." And he admitted, "I do not remember things now – I am getting old and going loopy."

But all day long he kept looking out of the window for his sister, telling me, "She is in this area."

Every hour of the day he will ask me, "What day is it today? Have I got anything to do today?"

I tell him, "No, we can relax today. We have no appointments for you."

He will give a big sigh of relief, saying, "Oh, thank goodness for that." And I will settle him down with his book, hoping I can get on with my work. But it never works on the days that he is restless because he won't sit reading for long. He starts following me around the house asking me over and over again, till I get sick of repeating myself.

I have to leave the housework or whatever I was trying to do and pay attention to him to stop him being restless.

I had to take him to see another specialist because although he goes to the toilet, he sometimes is not quick enough and during the last month I had had to wash and change his trousers at least four times every day. I felt like a dried-out old washerwoman. I had been working non-stop at washing his trousers.

The specialist told me he would let him try a trial drug to see if it could be of any help to him because he will not have a catheter in – he always pulls them out.

After a month the drug worked – no more trousers to wash every day, no more extra workload. As if I did not have a heavy enough load to bear already! I could not thank that specialist enough. What would we do without their help? Thank God for people like him.

So now Francis was on two trial drugs besides all his other tablets. He takes so many! I'm surprised they work, but they do.

He went back to the stage where he searches through the house. He had been doing it for four weeks now and I would leave him to it. It stopped him pestering me and I could get on with whatever needed to be done.

One day he had been searching all morning – he only stopped to have his dinner, then as soon as he had eaten he started again – but by now he was getting quite annoyed with himself. He started shouting at me to find it for him, saying to me, "I cannot find it."

I thought, 'I'd better try to calm him before he starts throwing his clothes around,' so I asked him, "What are you looking for?"

He told me he could not find his wallet.

I felt in his pocket and pulled out his wallet, telling him, "What can we do with you? Look, it is here all the time in your pocket."

He got very angry, snatching it off me, saying, "That's not it."

I told him, "But you only have one and all your identification is in there."

He was gritting his teeth, telling me, "That looks like it, but it is not the one." And he couldn't explain to me what the one he wanted looked like.

I knew there was no way of pacifying him, so I said, "You are always putting your wallet in a safe place so you don't lose it. So don't worry, you will remember where you put it tomorrow."

He said, "Oh yes, you're right. I will find it tomorrow." But all afternoon he carried on searching.

Here we go again. I could not believe it was only a couple of months since we were celebrating because we had been told by his diabetic nurse that his levels had been so good that he was classed as pre-diabetic and would not have to go to so many clinics now. I was happy, thinking there would be fewer trips to the nurse, but it had not lasted long. Now he was back again and the nurse told me he had to go on medication, either tablets or insulin, because his levels were uncontrolled again; so now he is a diabetic. I had thought at the time it would not last, and once again I was right. But we have to be thankful for small mercies and I had to try to start thinking positively. The nurse told me not to give Francis any sugar, biscuits or milk and to prepare smaller portions of meals, etc.

Francis was listening to all this, and when we got outside he said to me, "So now you are going to starve me again – I cannot eat." He was looking at me and saying in a distressed voice, "And I am not allowed a sweet cup of tea."

I told him, "Don't worry – I will not stop your cup of tea at your age. We will just cut down a little to see if it helps you."

He said, "So you are going to starve me at my age!"

It was the first time he had admitted he was getting on in years.

I told him, "I have no intention of not giving you a sweet cup of tea, and I have no intention of starving you. I will give you smaller portions, but I will give you more throughout the day."

He was happy with that.

While we were waiting to see the nurse for a prescription Francis had all the patients laughing again. On the screen it was telling people not to become a couch potato and make sure they did plenty of exercise and keep cool and drink plenty of water because of the heat.

He shouted out to me, "I want a couch potato."

I tried explaining to him that it is not something you eat, that it means don't sit on the couch all day and do your exercises.

He carried on shouting, "I want a couch potato. I don't sit all day. I do my walking. I want a couch potato – I will buy one myself."

BEFORE TIME SLIPS AWAY

Time goes by so quickly –
Enjoy time while you may.
There might not be another tomorrow,
There might not be another day,
Before time slips away.

Time goes by so quickly –
If a poor soul comes your way,
Help that soul do all you can

232

And you will be a wealthy man,
Not in money, only in kind,
Giving to you peace of mind
Before time slips away.

Time goes by so quickly –
There might come a time when you could be
A poor soul the same as he,
Needing help along your way,
Hoping someone comes to stay
To help you have a better day
Before time slips away.

Time goes by so quickly –
Time is great for all who care,
Make the most of it while it's there.
Try to do good, always be kind,
Love and happiness you will find
Staying with you day by day
Before time slips away.

Time goes by so quickly –
Enjoy time while you may.
There might not be another tomorrow,
There might not be another day,
Before time slips away.

All summer we had been to the park twice a week. It calms
Francis down when he starts to get anxious and annoyed
with himself. We always feed the ducks bread and mixed
seed. They love it and they know us by now. They spot us
coming and make a beeline straight for us, quacking away
and waggling their tails. They come out of the water and go
straight to Francis and take food straight out of his hand.

One duck, a black one, grabbed a full round out of his hand
before he had time to break it up, then it ran like the clappers
with it hanging from its mouth, hoping to reach the pond with

it, but the other ducks went legging after it. Before it had the chance to jump in the pond with it they grabbed it out of its mouth. Then it came back, waddling up to Francis, looking so forlorn and unhappy, staring up at him as if to say, "They have taken my bread off me – stolen it out of my mouth." He gave it another round of bread and it dashed through his legs, running under his wheelchair with it for protection, and then gobbled it up and came back from under his chair waggling its tail and looking at him as though quite proud of itself because it hads managed to keep it for itself. Then it flew on to the bench so it could get nearer to him.

Francis always recognises that duck because it is black. He always calls it Blackie and he always says to me, "Look, my friend Blackie has come to see me."

When we are leaving, Blackie swims away, but it always looks back and quacks as if to say goodbye and he always waves to it, saying, "Goodbye, Blackie, and thank you," which is what he says to our children when they have been to visit us. As they leave he goes to shake their hands and says, "Goodbye and thank you."

But our two daughters won't let him get away with that. They always say, "We don't want a handshake, we want a hug." And they grab hold of him and give him a hug. It is a good thing they know him and understand that he does not know who they are part of the time, but I can see it still upsets them.

I ask myself why Francis is always searching for things that are not there, things he will never find, and getting upset, annoyed and angry with himself when he finds nothing. I tell myself it is because he knows there is something wrong with his mind; he knows his mind has lost things, and he knows he cannot find what his mind has lost. He cannot bring them back. He tries fighting it, and he knows he is fighting a losing battle, but he won't give in. So he carries on searching like a lost, frightened soul, not knowing there is nothing he can do. I tell him he has dementia and it is a sickness that makes him forget things, and he will accept that. I tell him that is why he takes his tablets – because he is a poorly man – and he thanks me for helping him, but it does not stop him searching for what he has lost.

I watched the dementia slowly taking away everything from him a piece at a time. The first thing it took from him we will call stage one, which was his ability to mend things. He would try and try to fix things around the house, which he used to do without any problems, but he could not figure out how to mend things. No matter how hard he tried, he would always end up destroying or breaking whatever it was he attempted to mend – even simple things like plugs. It took him and me a year before we realised he was incapable, because I was always making excuses for him until in the end I could see it would be dangerous for both of us if I let him carry on. Even he admitted he could not fix things any more, so I stopped him trying and he told me he could not think clearly. But he did not like not fixing things for me – he would make that very clear – and I could not blame him, because what man wants to admit he cannot do the simplest of things around his own home? But he had destroyed so many things in the home that were not even broken before he had tried to mend them.

The arguments we had over stopping him were not very nice for me because I felt guilty. I felt as if I was trying to stop him being a man. In the end he stopped trying. Dementia had taken away his ability to think things out – stage one.

Stage two was when his memories slowly went away from him. Every holiday that we spent together has been wiped from his mind altogether. They are completely gone, never returning, lost forever. Gone are the wonders that we have seen together. Getting engaged, getting married – nothing brings these memories back to him, not even for one moment. Even looking at wedding photographs gives him no recollection whatever. Not even for one moment does anything come back to his mind. I talk to him to try and help him remember, but nothing!

I say, "Can you remember the time we saw your cousin in

Australia and we went swimming with her on the beach and the waves sent you sprawling all over the sand? You could not keep on your feet."

I would wait and hope that something would help him to remember, but I knew nothing would. It was not just him who had lost something; I felt like I had lost nearly everything too. So that's another thing he goes searching for: his memories – stage two.

In stage three older memories were wiped from his mind, lost. His own mother, sisters and brothers – I found out they were gone from his mind when I told him one of his sisters was coming to see him.

He said, "What are you talking about, sisters? I have no sisters. Are you going loopy? I don't know what you mean."

Then I told him about his mother and the rest of his family, telling him their names, but he told me, "You are loopy!"

So I asked him if he remembered his first wife, whom he had been married to for twenty years, and his son (who both tragically died in the 1980s). I was hoping he would remember them, but he stared at me, saying, "Now I know you are going loopy."

So I left well alone. No matter what I said or did to try and help him remember his mother and brothers and sisters I made no headway. Even showing him their photographs was futile. I felt deep sorrow for him. I hope that I never forget my mother and family, God willing. I tried to remind him of his family on many occasions afterwards, but nothing! His family were gone – stage three.

In stage four he began to lose his ability to communicate. I tried talking to him about what he used to do, but to everything I asked him I would get the same response: "I don't know. I cannot think. I cannot remember."

He could not respond to me when I tried to involve him in my interests. He would just sit there looking quite perplexed, never attempting to join in, never interested.

I gave him a notepad and pen, telling him to write a note to his grandchildren, asking them if he could go to their party.

He said, "Yes, I can do that."

He sat there for ages and I could see by his face he was trying to think what to write. He kept putting the pen to the pad, then hesitating, looking up and looking at me, so confused. I told him what to write down and he said, "Oh yes!" and put the pen to the pad again.

I thought, 'Good – he is writing something down.'

But then he looked around, looking up, puzzled.

After a while I asked him, "Have you finished writing, then?"

He said yes and gave me the pad.

I looked at what he had written, and there were a few scribbly lines, but nothing I could read.

When I take him visiting he never says one word to anyone. When they say something to him he will nod his head up and down as if he has understood what they are saying, but I can tell by the distant look on his face that he does not know what they are on about.

He will sit there and every so often he will say, "Fine day, is it not?" He will keep repeating that over and over again while we are talking. After he has said it he will smile, thinking he is holding a conversation with them. And I suppose he is in his own way – the only way he can.

Then when we have to leave he shakes their hands as if they are strangers.

Before his sickness he was a right chatterbox, always on about fishing, sailing or shooting. He was always writing things down. He never went anywhere without his writing book and pen. He was always drawing maps showing where he would be going. Now he has lost the ability to communicate or correspond with his own family or me, his wife, or even himself – stage four.

In stage five he lost his home. I found out he had lost his home one day when he had gone for his usual walk. Before that day he would walk down the drive, go out of the gate, pass two houses, then turn around and come straight to his own gate and back into the house. That was as far as he could manage to walk, then he would have to rest for a while. He would have no problem about finding his own home. This time he did not turn around! I always watched him when he went for his walk because in one of the different phases he went through he would be liable to wander away.

So when he didn't turn back I ran after him, asking him, "Where are you going?"

He was in a very distressed state, white-faced and waving his arms in the air, saying, "I cannot find my home. I don't know where it is. I don't know where I live. It was here before, but now it has gone. Where is my home?"

I turned him around and took him home. He walked around the house, trying to recognise things, but he could not. I could not make him see he was home. Ever since then he searches for his home – stage five.

In stage six he is slowly losing his wife, his stepchildren, grandchildren and great-grandchildren. He would forget who we were but we'd always come back to his mind; then the memory wouldn't come back for up to two months: then it was six months and now he has not remembered me, his wife, for a full year. He has always called me by my name – he has never forgotten my name – but I am just a carer, someone who takes care of his daily needs.

When I ask him, "Who do you think I am?"

He always says, "I don't know who you are, but you are Iris."

So I get a bit of solace out of that because up to now he still remembers my name.

When he sees and studies the grandchildren's photographs on the wall he will always ask, "Who are them children?" I tell him and he says, "Oh yes!" But I know he does not remember, for if he had remembered them he would not have asked.

But when they come to see him or if we go to see them he is so very happy. They give him great joy, so we always look forward to that.

I hate it when we are sat together at night and he gets up and looks out of the window, searching for his wife. Gone are his treasured possessions, wife and children – stage six.

Every morning when he awakes he always says, "Good morning. It is a nice day today." Even though sometimes it is winter and blowing a gale outside, every morning is the same. He has never missed one morning in all the seventeen years I have known him, and up to now the dementia has not stopped him saying it. When he says it every day I always think to myself, 'I hope it will be a nice day today.' These this last few months he has had more bad days than good.

Before he goes to sleep at night, regardless if he sleeps or not, he will always say, "Night night. God bless. I love you." That is another thing that he still says, no matter what, and I hope the dementia never takes those few words away from him and me, because after a hard day of running after him, at his beck and call, those few words he says to me morning and night make me feel happy and good and make everything I do worthwhile. I feel like I have something left, because sometimes I feel empty and so lonely.

The mental-health psychiatrist consultant tested him again to find out how he was progressing because his last scan showed abnormal cells, so he had another scan because his body jumps every hour of the night and to me he looked like a man with Parkinson's. But when he got the results of the scan Francis did not have anything other than vascular dementia.

The psychiatrist told me Francis can understand what is being told to him, but cannot retain it at all.

I thought, 'Tell me something new!'

I had to take him to my friend's birthday party – the friend who likes to make him blush. He did not want to go – isn't it funny that he remembers she is the one who embarrasses him! But I managed to get him there in the end. I kept telling him if he does not want to stay, if he becomes tired, then I will bring him straight back home. He had been moaning all day long with his aches and pains, so I was happy to get out and about. My friend had threatened me: if I did not take him, she would come to my house and take him and leave me behind. So I thought I would go just for one hour.

I was glad I took him. He really enjoyed himself. He was singing away with everybody, even though he was not singing what they were. It was nice to see him trying to sing and clapping his hands and smiling away. He even had a tot of whisky, which he enjoyed. I was happy I took him. I was only going to stay for one hour, but we stayed till midnight, which was five hours.

That night he slept all through, which meant it was the most sleep I had had for a long time, and he did not get up till 9 a.m.

I thought to myself, 'It is a pity we cannot have a party and a tot of whisky every night.' He never complained all the time he was there, and his aches and pains miraculously disappeared, but I'm afraid if we did too much partying I know it would see him off. But what is that old saying – 'What a way to go!'

He was on about it all the next day, saying how he loved going to her party.

I told him, "Yes, you enjoyed yourself, but it was only because she was too busy to try and make you blush. But don't worry, she will make it up to you when you see her again."

For a couple of months he was in the phase of wandering off, so I had to sleep on the door keys. I wonder if I put him in that frame of mind by saying I would take him round to my friend's house, because when she grabs his hand he goes deathly white and tries to get away. I thought I might have scared him so that all he can think of is getting as far away as possible, but no, it was probably not me as he always wanders off every so many months. He flits from one phase to another.

At one o'clock one morning it was pitch-black outside and pouring with rain. I woke up to him wandering around the bedroom. He was filling his pockets up with lots of things from his dresser drawers.

I asked him, "What are you doing?"

I got the same answer he always gives me when he is in the phase of wandering away, which is, "I am heading down south, then I will head east to the sea."

When I asked him, "Why? Where are you going?"

He said, "I don't know."

I told him, "Look, it's the middle of the night. Come back to bed and we can talk about it after a good night's sleep."

Thankfully he always agrees.

In the morning I empty his pockets and put the things he has stuffed in them back into his dresser drawers. That night there were two pairs of glasses, his razor, a wallet, a comb, a handkerchief and two tubes of antiseptic cream. He had never put the cream in his pockets before – his toes must have been playing him up!

While I was taking them out of his pockets he was watching me and he said, "What are you doing? Why is that lot in my coat?"

I told him, "I am turfing this lot out of your pockets and putting them back in your drawers because last night you were going down south again and you put this lot in your pockets."

He said, looking quite puzzled, "I must be going loopy. I don't remember doing that and I don't know anybody down south."

But I know years ago he used to work down south as a prison officer.

When he had finished his breakfast he kept insisting I give him the door key, and saying he must go down south! I told him that we only had the one and I would need it. He kept insisting I give it to him, getting so agitated, I told him I would take him shopping and I would get a key made for him. It calmed him down for a while, but I had to find ways and means of distracting his mind from wanting the door key for at least a month, until he moved on to his next phase, which was back to his searching.

He had been searching for things around the house for a week, and I had been ignoring him, letting him get on with it, then one day he would not leave me alone. I had bathed and helped him dress in his nightclothes, but he would not rest

241

and he would not let me ignore him. After he had followed me around and after he had pulled all the drawers out and flung everything on the floor I had had enough.

I asked him, "OK, just what is it you are looking for?"

He said, "The buckle for my dressing gown."

I told him that it did not have a buckle and I tied it for him. He settled down after that.

As I had ignored him, it serves me right.

After breakfast one day he said, "Right, can you take me to the bus stop?" I knew by the look on his face he was wanting to go away again. He was stood there waving his arm in the air, getting agitated. "Take me to the bus stop."

I told him, "You cannot go on a bus unless you know where you are going to."

He said, "I don't know where I am going to, but I am going on a bus."

I explained to him, "You are a very poorly man at the moment and you are not allowed on the bus. You must promise me you will not go away or go on a bus without me being with you."

He promised me he would not wander away without me, but all day he kept repeating to me, "Take me to the bus. I need to go on the bus."

I just kept on ignoring him.

One day he gave me something new. He said to me, "Merry Christmas!"

I said, "Oh, so it's Christmas in April now, is it?"

He said, "Yes, and I'd better have a shave or you may think I am Father Christmas."

All day he was in a happy mood and he kept on asking me what I wanted for a present. I could not shut him up and I did not want to tell him it was not Christmas, so I took him out shopping and let him buy me a present because he was so happy. He kept asking me what present I wanted.

I told him, "You can think of one – whatever you think I would like."

He said, "I will buy you a watch."

So I took him to the shop and he bought me a watch.

On the way back home he said to me, "I will tell my wife you are a good driver."

I said to him, "Will you tell your wife you gave me a present?"

He was looking bewildered, so I said, "Never mind – you can buy your wife some earrings. She will like that."

He was smiling and happy with that.

I thought to myself, 'I wonder who he thinks I really am.' I know he would miss me if I was not there. I think he knows I am family, but cannot remember which one. At least I know I am important to him and he needs me. At least while he stays like this he is manageable, but I know there will come a time when he becomes unmanageable. I will deal with that when it comes.

When he goes on his walks up the drive I can see he gets weaker by the day because every four steps he stops for a breather. At least when we stay in for the day he still does his walks without me having to force him to. I know that he knows he is getting weaker because sometimes I can see by his eyes that he has had a good cry, and, like me, a good cry does him the world of good.

One week I think he did most of his phases together. He did nothing else but ask me where his wife had gone and when was he going to her room? Then he went back to his army days, then he asked for his children, then he started searching for something. He does not know what he is searching for, but he never stops.

I think he's trying to find anything – anything he can hang on to, anything that will stay with him, anything he cannot lose. It's no good me trying to help, I have tried so many times and it does not help him one bit. It is like telling a child to behave itself – it just falls on deaf ears. I have to leave him till each phase has passed.

LIFE

Compare life with water and sand
Forever running through your hand.
We grasp hold of it to make it stay
For it to only slip away.
Life is not here for very long –
No sooner here than it is gone.

Each of us has a road to travel too –
Each of us must see it through.
So many hills we have to climb,
Which takes us through a length of time.
All of us have a heart that is free;
None of us know our destiny.

Life passes on from you and me.
It is only then that we do see
Life comes from woman, life comes from man
To stay on Earth for as long as it can.
Life is precious, but it does not stay –
Life comes and goes from day to day.

As we go along a very hard road,
Some carrying a heavy load,
A turning point we hope to find,
Hoping for a good life in our mind,
Never stopping to wonder why,
Life coming, life going, passing on by.
Compare life with water and sand
Forever running through your hand.
We grasp hold of it to make it stay
For it to only slip away.
Life is not here for very long –
No sooner here than it is gone.

Francis always drags his left leg when he walks. I tell him to bend his knee, but he never does.

I tell him, "You walk like a lame horse, and if you were a horse you would have been shot by now." Or I say, "Apart from the way you walk, always with a stiff dragging leg, you remind me of a zombie – you remind me of the walking dead."

He will laugh about it, and it is a good job he has a sense of humour. On a good day he will say, "OK, well, this zombie wants a cup of tea."

So I will tell him, "Oh yes, well, get off your backside and get it yourself because you're not dead yet, even though you look it and sometimes act it. I could hire you out for Halloween."

It was another visit to the hospital again after another fall. That was five times he had fallen in one year. I was hoping he didn't have another bleed in his eyes, because last time that happened he had laser treatment on it and we were going to hospital appointments for a full year. This time he was lucky. After they photographed his eyes we knew he had done no damage and we only got an appointment for a check-up in six months' time. That was all right by him – he loves appointments because he always thinks he is going on holiday, and in his mind he is.

My friends always say to me, "I don't know how you stand it because he is always sick – it never stops."

I tell them, "I'm used to it by now. Everybody gets sick at some time in their life, and if they didn't then they should be thankful for their health and live life to the full and make the best of it. He might be always sick, but at least it does not stop him from living life as best he can. Plus he is very happy. On his good days he still finds things I say to him humorous and he knows he can say what he likes to me without either of us taking it to heart. When I call him a zombie he laughs and smiles and tries to say something back that is funny. He cannot usually think of anything, but whatever he says I make out it was funny and it lifts his spirits, especially when I tell him not to run away and leave me or I will send the police after him. That makes him smile."

Occasionally he fell out of the bed. When he does that he does not hurt himself because there is a large thick rug for him to fall on and nothing in his way to catch himself on – or so I thought. One night the door was slightly open and he caught himself on the catch near the handle of the door (I have removed the catch now so such a freak accident cannot happen again).

I lifted him back on to the bed, and when I checked him over I realised he was bleeding all over the sheets and blanket. I found the door catch had left a cut on his face from his ear to his mouth. It was not deep, but because he is on warfarin (anticoagulant treatment) he bleeds a lot. I had to put pressure on the wound, clean it with Dettol, then put wound-healing ointment on it. That did it. I always keep a tube of that handy for him – it puts a film over the cut. The bed looked like a murder had been committed, but the wound healed up after a couple of days.

I took him to be checked over and told the doctor about his fall. He recommended rehab for him at a 'falls clinic'. He loved it and so did I. The bus would pick him up right outside our door, and someone would be with him at all times. He was monitored to see what he could or could not do and they taught him how to walk more steadily and how to get up and down without losing his balance. With his sickness he could not do much, but it was exercise for him to stop his muscles seizing up. He went twice a week – Tuesday and Friday from nine to twelve.

I had never had so much respite! I must say I really enjoyed it and they were so good to him.

Now I take him every Friday for just two hours – it helps keep him moving – and I have got him a small foot cycle, which he uses for just five minutes at a time on his good days. Plus he still takes his walks up the drive. Sometimes I tell him he is fitter than me.

Everyone admires the way he gets on with what he does.

I have to be so careful when I hide the door key. I only keep one for me and my daughter keeps one, but for all his forgetfulness Francis is so crafty. He watches me to see where I hide it. At night-time I sleep with it under my pillow, and in the daytime I keep it in my cardigan pocket. This day – his great escape day – was so hot, so I took my cardigan off, leaving the door key in the pocket, and hung it on the bedroom door. He was supposedly in the living room, quietly reading his book, quite unconcerned about what I was doing. Well, that is what I thought.

I was hanging out the washing and I thought I heard someone at my front door, so I went to look. It was open. Then I realised Francis had got my key and was gone. I ran down the street hoping to catch him, hoping he had not gone far. I was thinking to myself, 'If he has gone too far down I will go back for the car and search the streets for him before I put out a search party.'

I saw him as I turned the corner – I could not believe my eyes! He was nearly at the other end of the street, running like the clappers, and him supposedly a cripple needing my help to lift him up and down.

I was absolutely shattered trying to catch up with him, but I thought to myself, 'I have to keep him in my sight because he could disappear easily in this area.'

We are surrounded by fields and if he had headed into those he would have been in trouble. He only had trousers and a light T-shirt on. I was trying to catch him and shouting his name at the top of my voice. At one point he even turned round, and I'm sure he saw me and heard me shouting, but he carried on. He was actually sprinting along and putting me to shame, because I was the one who was supposed to be fitter than him and here I was trying my best to keep up with him.

I caught up with him and grabbed hold of his shirt, and it was a while before I could speak. I was breathless, but he was all right. He was trying to take my hands off his shirt to get me off him so that he could get away.

I kept trying to turn him around, all the time saying, "Where are you going? Your home is this way. Come back home with me."

He was still trying to get my hands off him, thrashing around, getting mad and defensive with me. He had escaped and did not want to go back. He was a free man. I tried talking softly to him, pleading with his better nature, trying to soothe him.

He stopped trying to push me away from him and started walking back with me.

When we got back to a few doors away from our house he pointed to a parked car and started running towards it in an angry manner, shouting out, "That is my car! They have stolen it away from me." He was trying to open the car door saying, "It is my car! They have taken it away from my area."

I got hold of him and said in a stern and angry voice, "Look, if you touch that car again they will bring the police to us because it is not your car. You're not allowed a car – you are too sick to drive. You are a poorly man. Come back home with me and we can talk it over before the police come. Otherwise you will get into trouble."

He reluctantly walked back home with me, and I managed to calm him down. Every so often he would look out of the window and say, "They have stolen my car from my area."

I found my door key on the drive and thought to myself, 'I shall have to keep it round my neck on a chain or something. I am not a miracle worker. I cannot keep a dog collar on him, although judging by that escape I think he needs one.'

So every day I make sure he has his key ring on him, which tells people to look in his pocket for his credentials. I must make sure he carries them at all times, because obviously he will try to escape again at some time or other.

I asked him, "What were you running away from? Are you not happy with me? Am I that frightening?"

He just laughed. He did not know what I was on about.

I could not sleep one night because he was in and out of the bed. I usually keep putting him back to bed, but this time I pretended to be asleep. I was curious to see just what he was up to. I always sleep on the door key, so I thought, 'He cannot get out, so I will see what he gets up to. I will let him get on with whatever he wants to do. He won't let me sleep, but at least I am here resting.'

He went out of the bedroom, just wandering around, looking lost. Then he got back into bed. After he had five minutes' sleep he got out of bed and checked the time on his watch (which he had put on the last time he got out of bed). Then he got a bag out of the drawer and put his razor and comb in it. Then he got his shoes and wrapped the shoes and bag in one of his thick woollen jumpers, twirling them round to keep them tightly together. He stood there nodding his head up and down with satisfaction, then put them on a chair on the other side of the bedroom. He patted his belly, then he put his hat and coat on over his nightclothes and started filling up his pockets with lots of things from out of the drawers until his pockets were bulging. He tried for about ten minutes to fasten up his coat, but could not manage it. He looked around the bedroom, checked the jumper and shoes were safe on the chair, patted his belly again, checked his watch, then got back into bed and slept for ten minutes. Then he sat up in bed, looking across at the jumper with his shoes wrapped in it. He moved his head up and down with satisfaction, checked his watch, then slept again. He kept repeating the same actions all night.

I don't know how he slept with all that stuff in his pockets, but he did. It did not seem to worry him.

If I lie on a crease in the sheet I cannot sleep. It annoys me.

I felt pity and sorrow for Francis, watching him do those things. I kept thinking I should take the stuff out of his pockets, but he would only have filled them up again and he was happy doing what he was doing. I did not really want to intrude on him, and I managed to get a bit of rest.

In the morning when I got up to make his breakfast he said to me, "What time did we land?"

I looked at the clock and said, "Eight o'clock!"

He smiled at me saying, "Oh, good. When are we driving home?"

I said, "It is OK, we are already home, so put your gear away while I make breakfast."

He went and emptied his pockets, took his hat and coat off and sat down, smiling and eating his breakfast.

I thought to myself, 'I am glad I let him carry on with what he thought he should be doing, without me interrupting him all the time.' So I decided that in the future I would just go along with it and leave him to it because it makes him happy and he is hurting nobody. If I stop him he will think I am taking things away from him; I would be robbing him of his fantasies, robbing him of his holidays, and over the years dementia has done enough of that.

It was bedtime, and I had just got ready for bed when he said to me, "Come on, then, are you ready for the run?"

I answered, "What run is that, then?"

He said, "You know, we have to run with all the runners." And he started dragging me towards the front door.

It took me all my time not to laugh. I told him, "What, me run with a load of runners? I don't think I could manage to run down the garden path. And come to that, you cannot even walk down it."

He was quite determined, still trying to drag me to the door for this run, saying, "Come on, we have to join the runners."

I had to try and calm him. I said, "OK, I will go on the run with you if you show me how. You can demonstrate a practice run to show me how to do it."

He smiled and said, "OK, it's easy."

He stopped trying to drag me and stood there with one foot in front of him and one hand stretched out in front with his other hand behind him. It was a good stance. It would have put anyone to shame. At least he looked like a runner, if nothing else. I stood waiting to catch him because I knew he would fall, but I had to let him have a go because he would not give in. It was the only way I could bring him back to reality and shut him up.

He stood on the spot and said, "One, two, three."

I did not think he could still count.

When he tried to run, he took one step and lost his balance, falling straight on to me. I managed to keep him upright, which was hard because he is so heavy.

Then I told him with a stern voice, "There you are! I told you you could not run. If I had not caught you you would have fallen down again, and then I would have had to take you to hospital once again."

He was a bit shaken up, but I could not get that stance he did out of my mind. I started laughing, which made him laugh – he looked so funny.

I told him in between laughing, "It is a good job you don't have to go on any run, because judging by what you just showed me I think we both need to practise first."

He said to me, "I did not know that I could not run."

I said, "Well, maybe you will take more notice of me in the future."

I always try to turn the things he does and says into a laugh. I have learnt to just go along with him because I cannot bring him back to reality however much I try to do so. If he thinks he is on holiday, so be it. He is enjoying himself and he thinks I am with him. I will tell him I am enjoying it too. It is best that way, because then I can get on with what I need to do in peace. If anything he says hurts me I know it can be dismissed from my mind, because I know he does not know what he is saying. It is his dementia talking, not him.

Now I always try positive thinking; any other way just makes my life a misery. Who wants that? I have to try to be strong for the both of us, and let nothing play on my mind. Being weak does not solve anything.

I wait to see what phase is coming next. He goes in and out of them like stepping stones. I usually know what's coming next: he is either on his holidays, in the army, wandering off, searching around, losing his wife and children, losing his home and his possessions, catching aeroplanes, catching buses or going to the sea, going to the south. He is always trying to escape from something, especially me.

I know all his phases. I learnt them along the way – the hard way. Dementia not only took everything from him; it took everything from me. Yes, I still have him, but he is only the shell of the man he used to be. But he is still with me. After what he has been through I think he is my Superman, even though I call him my zombie.

We still get out and about, some poor devils cannot even do that, so we have a lot to be thankful for. Nobody knows what it is like living with somebody who has dementia until they go through it, night after night, day after day, year after year, living with it. And if dementia alone is not bad enough, throw in many other ailments and sicknesses for good luck. At least I know he is thankful for everything I have done for him – committing my life to him, trying to keep him safe and happy, always trying to be kind and helpful, because after everything I do for him he never misses saying the two words that make it all worthwhile, which are 'thank you'.

In sickness and health, until death us do part.

FOREVER TAKE MY HAND

Take my hand, I will help you.
Swallow all your pride.
No matter what you say or do
I will stay by your side.
Forever take my hand.

Sometimes there is happiness,
Sometimes there is pain.
Accept my helping hand,
With you I shall remain.
Forever take my hand.

When the sun is shining
We feel happy, we feel glad.
When it starts to rain
We feel miserable and sad.
Forever take my hand.

Come rain or shine, no matter what,
I will be with you all the time.
We will forever have a bond,
Everything will turn out fine.
Forever take my hand.

Have trust and faith in me –
I shall forever be around.
Have confidence and you will see
I shall never let you down.
Forever take my hand.

Take my hand, I will help you.
Swallow all your pride.
No matter what you say or do
I will stay by your side.
Forever take my hand.

THREE STARS

I have three stars locked in my heart,
Each one plays a special part.
One at a time I pass to you
So you can pass each one on too.

The first star is love.
Once in love, never to part,
Given to someone you adore,
A feeling you would die for,
A feeling deep within the heart –
Love.

The second star is kindness.
Help the poor who pass your way
So they can live through another day.
Soothe them when they're showing fear,
Stay beside them to show you care –
Kindness.

The third star is hope.
Put others first, help them cope,
Talk with them, give them hope,
Help them when they have lost their way,
Help them think positive every day –
Hope.